W0246801

Gender, Medicine, and Society in Colonial India

Gender, Medicine, and Society in Colonial India

Women's Health Care in Nineteenth- and Early Twentieth-Century Bengal

Sujata Mukherjee

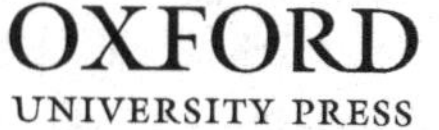
OXFORD
UNIVERSITY PRESS

OXFORD
UNIVERSITY PRESS

Oxford University Press is a department of the University of Oxford. It furthers the University's objective of excellence in research, scholarship, and education by publishing worldwide. Oxford is a registered trademark of Oxford University Press in the UK and in certain other countries.

Published in India by
Oxford University Press
YMCA Library Building, 1 Jai Singh Road, New Delhi 110 001, India

First Edition published in 2017

ISBN-13: 978-0-19-946822-5
ISBN-10: 0-19-946822-2

Typeset in Adobe Jenson Pro 10.7/13.3
by Tranistics Data Technologies, Kolkata 700 091
Printed in India by Replika Press Pvt. Ltd

For Ma, Baba, and Tanya

Contents

Acknowledgements

This book represents many years of thinking and research on a topic that I find fascinating. I have incurred many debts in the course of researching and writing this book.

Over the years, I have benefitted from the help and advice rendered by friends and colleagues and the untiring services of librarians and archivists who helped me locate my sources.

I am especially indebted to the librarians and custodians of the National Library, Kolkata; the Nehru Memorial Museum and Library, New Delhi; the National Archives of India, New Delhi; the Directorate of State Archives, Kolkata; Bangiya Sahitya Parishat, Kolkata; Ramakrishna Mission Institute of Culture, Kolkata; Centre for Studies in Social Sciences, Kolkata; the central library at Visva-Bharati, Bolpur; the libarary at Rabindra Bharati University, Kolkata; and the library at the Institute of Development Studies, Kolkata (IDSK).

I am deeply indebted to Professor Amiya Kumar Bagchi, Professor Achin Chakraborty, and Dr Ramkrishna Chatterjee of IDSK for a fellowship at the Rabindranath Tagore Centre for Human Development Studies (RTCHDS)—a joint initiative of the IDSK and the University of Calcutta—during 2011–12, and to the authorities of the Rabindra Bharati University for granting me lien during that period. The help and stimulus provided by the staff and faculty of the IDSK and the extraordinarily congenial environment of the Institute made possible a year of uninterrupted work on this project.

I have immensely benefitted from discussions with my colleagues at the Department of History, Rabindra Bharati University, over the years, including with Professor Tripti Chaudhuri, Professor Himadri Banerjee, Dr Rajsekhar Basu, Dr Sanjukta Das Gupta, Professor Srilata Chatterjee, Professor Susnata Das, Dr Ashis Das, Dr Hitendra Kumar Patel, Dr Anuradha Kayal, Dr Sahara Ahmed, and Dr Ajanta Biswas. I am also indebted to my friends and colleagues at Calcutta University, Jadavpur University, Kolkata, Burdwan University, Vidyasagar University, Medinipur, and Visva-Bharati, who invited me over the years for special lectures, talks, and seminar presentations, which gave me opportunities for discussing and sharing many of my ideas and research findings. I am especially indebted to Professor Deepak Kumar and also Professor Chittabrata Palit for their comments and invaluable suggestions. The days I spent as a visiting scholar at the Zakir Husain Centre for Educational Studies in Jawaharlal Nehru University, New Delhi, at the Indian Institute of Science, Bengaluru (Centre for Contemporary Studies), and as visiting ICCR Chair at the Wellington University, New Zealand, also provided me with opportunities to discuss my ideas and interact with scholars, teachers, and students.

Professor Biswamoy Pati has offered informed and insightful suggestions for the improvement of early drafts and I am immensely grateful for his untiring support, patience, guidance, and encouragement. I am also thankful to Professor Sekhar Bandyopadhyay, Head of School, School of History, Philosophy, Political Science, and International Relations, Victoria University, Wellington, New Zealand, for his invaluable comments.

I am also grateful to two anonymous reviewers of the manuscript for their suggestions. Last but not the least, I am especially thankful to Oxford University Press for publishing this book.

Introduction

This book is about the convergence of medicine and gender in a colonial setting, intending to show how far and in what ways this convergence was important in different trajectories involved in the politics of health in the South Asian context. Over the last few years, scholars have become engaged in exploring the gender dimensions of the colonial space.[1]

Different studies published so far on the interrelated theme of gender and medicine in colonial India, as well as those on different aspects of disease, medicine, and health care, have thrown light on some of the aspects with a bearing on women's health. These include studies on the work of medical missionaries in the sphere of Indian women's health care, medicalization of childbirth, politics of reproductive health, growth of medical education and profession for women, careers of female practitioners of indigenous medicine, curative facilities for female patients in hospitals and asylums, and involvement of British women in designing health care for women of India. The history of mental health of

European women and the history of asylums have also received some amount of scholarly attention.[2]

In the context of colonial Bengal, the issues of medical education and medical profession for women as well as aspects of reproductive health have so far claimed some amount of research attention. It will not be unreasonable to assume that the fact that the involvement of the colonial state in the matter of health care for women remained only minimal[3] worked as a deterrent to take up any full-scale study dealing with gender and medicine till date. Yet no one can deny that in the history of two hundred years of colonial rule, crucial developments in the discursive as well as empirical fields of medicine and health care touched the lives of women in significant ways, and that gender and politics of medicine contributed in multiple ways in formulating perceptions and identities at the intersection of colonialism, class, caste, communities, and nation. Thus, studies in the social history of medicine remain incomplete without an attempt to analyse different slippages between medicine and gender. In order to contribute towards an understanding of multiple axes through which gender operated in colonial medicine, my work intends to contextualize multiple features of broad changes in the arena of health and medicine in British Bengal with any relation to women—be it growth of different curative institutions or foundation of educational establishments, reform of midwifery, discourses on sexuality, marriage reforms, birth control, the voluntary sector's involvement in the delivery of health care, evolution of public health administration, growth of nationalist politics, or emergence of women's associations in the late colonial period—each of which remained in different degrees crucial in the politics of gender and medicine throughout the colonial period.

Colonial Medicine

As is well known, Western medicine, introduced by the British in India, could never accomplish the task of replacing indigenous medical systems or of providing cure for any significant size of the population even by the end of the colonial rule. One major importance of Western medicine lay in the role it played in the process of colonization, acting as an ideological as well as empirical 'tool of empire'.[4] According to David Arnold, 'Colonialism used—or attempted to use—the body as a site for the construction of its own authority, legitimacy, and control. In part, therefore, the history of colonial medicine, and of the epidemic diseases with which it was so closely entwined, serves to illustrate the more general nature of colonial power and knowledge and to illuminate its hegemonic as well as its coercive processes.'[5]

History of Western medicine in the colonial context is, however, no longer limited to the interpretation of it acting as a tool of empire, which had earlier dominated the works of scholars like Daniel Headrick and Philip Curtin. Since the early 1980s, discussions focusing on the question of what is colonial about colonial medicine—originally analysed by Roy Porter and later rearticulated by Shula Marks—became important.[6] The 1990s saw a great deal of path-breaking studies attempting to expose the complex history of Western medicine in colonial settings, including India and Africa. Waltraud Ernst, in her book *Mad Tales from the Raj*, has discussed the 'politics of control'.[7] David Arnold, in his pioneering work *Colonizing the Body*, published in 1993, points out that 'Western medicine was intimately bound up with the nature and aspirations of the colonial state itself'.[8] He even argues that the case of India demonstrates 'in a manner unparalleled in Western societies, the exceptional importance of medicine in the cultural and political constitution of its subjects'.[9]

While recognizing his indebtedness to Michel Foucault, Arnold, however, points out at the same time that he attempts to study the creation of a state-centred system of scientific knowledge and power, rather than the 'more diffused and generalized forms of knowledge and power' described by Foucault. He also claims that in his analysis, seeing the question of resistance as an essential element in the evolution and articulation of a particular system of medical thought and action constitutes another major point of departure from Foucault's work.

Mark Harrison's *Public Health in British India*, published in 1994, explores the theoretical, professional, and administrative aspects of the development of public health in British India, thereby privileging colonial medical administration.[10] His work also delineates the importance of studying the agency and identity of Anglo-Indian preventive medicine. Both Arnold and Harrison devote considerable attention to the work of an Indian scholar of modern medicine in colonial India, Radhika Ramasubban. In Radhika Ramasubban's publications, the medical establishment of British India is characterized as overridingly concerned with maintaining the health of Europeans in their colonial enclaves, and particularly with preserving the health of the army.[11]

In some of the recent writings on the history of colonial medicine in India, historians have emphasized the necessity of recognizing that the domination of the knowledge of Western medicine in the colonies passed through various stages and that there was a greater degree of dialogue in the sphere of production of knowledge in the colonies than is usually recognized.[12]

It has been stated by several scholars that 'colonial medicine' is related to a larger quest, similar to the concern expressed in postcolonial history writing: 'Is there a difference between the colonial state and the modern state in Europe?'[13] The colonial state has in fact been identified by some as a modern, biopolitical one where the concept of race was deployed as a scientific ideology. Medicine, in its turn, as a crucial ideology of the (liberal) empire, served to produce and disseminate ideas of race in such a way that race appeared as one of the normalizing strategies of the modern biopolitical state. Ann Laura Stoler has even gone so far as to suggest that no historical context is more fruitful for an examination of a biopolitical state than the colonial one. According to Stoler, race and colonialism were fundamental to modern discourses on sex and selfhood, and the construction of identity markers of race, sex, culture, and class in fact flowed back and forth between the metropole and the colony. She points out that disciplinary categories and bodily tactics invented in one part of the colonial world were used in another in the formulation of private and public selves.[14] To comprehend the colonial processes that created modern subjects and subjectivities, she suggests that we move beyond the cordon sanitaire of medical discourse and study intimate and everyday aspects of the lives of the colonized—the toilet, the diet, the bedroom, and so on. About the process of subjectification under colonial rule, Gyan Prakash raised a debatable issue by stating: 'To govern Indians as modern subjects required colonial knowledge and colonial regulation to function as self-knowledge and self-regulation, but this was impossible under colonialism.'[15] According to Prakash, in the colony, the practices of modern government—sanitation, the control of epidemics, the establishment of colonial institutions—had to operate as acts of colonial rule, and therefore, presumably, they failed to fulfil their 'normalizing' functions. Prakash's thesis of impossibility has been questioned by other scholars. It has been pointed out that some of the practices such as sanitation did operate as 'acts of colonial rule' but certain other practices such as regulation of hygienic behaviour were disseminated as norms of self-government and also used by sections of the native population as tactics of self-regulation and self-knowledge.[16] It has been pointed out that by analysing 'the ways in which the disciplines (an anatomo-politics of the human body) worked with regulatory controls (a biopolitics of the population)' and also by recognizing 'the role of biopower (those diverse techniques for achieving the subjugation of bodies and control of populations) in the universalization of difference', it would be possible to push beyond the Said-inflected critique of colonial power/knowledge and adopt what might be termed a late-Foucauldian approach to the colonial medical archive.[17] In this genre of analysis, convergence of liberalism, or 'a science of empire' and colonial medicine, or 'an empire of science' meant recognizing 'race' to be serving as a post-enlightenment, modern ideology—based on principles and methods relating to science, nature, biology, and evolution. Thus, colonial India was not only influenced by race science in Europe, as suggested by David Arnold, but was a constitutive of race science.[18] It has been argued that 'a racially grounded medicine served to extend colonial power, just as it created the modern subject of colonialism'.[19] From yet another point of view, new perceptions have led scholars to look beyond the realm of state medicine and adopt new approaches to study the colonial medical archive. Prajit Bihari Mukharji focuses on *daktari* medicine or vernacularization of Western medicine through the exposition of medicine by practising doctors in colonial Bengal. He unpacks the political process of establishing new hierarchies of power, and argues that pluralization of the knowledge of Western medicine would entail 'a parallel pluralisation of modernity itself', because 'Western' medicine was a crucial component of the project of colonial modernity.[20]

The view of medical anthropologists that the idea of healing is representative of a cultural system or process that shaped social change also seems to strengthen the idea of medical pluralism. However, since this study belongs to the genre of social history of medicine, there is not much scope to explore that angle here. It is also important to remember that the analytical framework presented by scholars working on colonial locations other than India can be applied usefully for analysing changes in colonial scenarios elsewhere. Megan Vaughan, in her 1991 book *Curing Their Ills*, explicated how the terms 'African' and 'African illness' came to be produced through biomedical discourse. She points out that 'biomedicine is practiced and interpreted by African doctors, nurses and medical assistants and as a practice is therefore as "African" as any other healing system'.[21] According to some scholars, Vaughan's work represents a fruitful intervention in the analysis of colonial medicine in that 'it marks a shift from a focus on the operation of colonial power through medicine to an analysis of the constant articulation of colonial power on medical knowledge, and its respective relation to the "subject"'. She also points out that the aspect of productive capacity of power—as emphasized by Foucault in his analysis of modern power—has remained rather underutilized by historians of medicine, and that it would be more useful to focus on medicine's role not only exclusively in the process of objectification but also in how it entails creation of individuated subjects capable of self-making and control. At the same time, Vaughan is cautious to point out that in the colonial context, power's productive capacity for subjectification remains limited. Colonial power in Africa was different from the modern power because of the particular and uneven development of capitalism in that context. She also suggests, like Arnold, that there is no possibility of any effective resistance to power within a Foucauldian world view, since the discourses of resistance are themselves permeated with the very ideas of freedom and liberation which constitute the modern power/knowledge regime. Colonialist discourse, as shown by scholars, sought patholization of colonial subjects through medicine in order to naturalize and rationalize otherness. Sander Gilman has demonstrated how nineteenth-century discourses were marked by slippages between race, gender, and class.[22]

Vaughan, on her part, highlights the organization of racial, gendered, and other differences on a universal scheme of things via the discursive domains of medicine. Moreover, she states two vital points: first, medicine did not always gender its colonial subjects in any direct way, and second, that the gendering of colonial subjects cannot be assumed to be monolithic.

An observation made by Shula Marks is also noteworthy in this connection. She writes: 'Western biomedicine has undoubtedly played a major role, both in making universalizing claims, and in creating and reproducing racial and gendered discourses of difference.'[23]

Gender and Colonial Medicine

Both the aspects of the processes of objectification and subjectification served through medicine in the realm of gender in colonial India are sought to be highlighted in this book. The underlying attempt is to explore the slippages between race, gender, and class in the working of medicine in colonial India. In other words, this work supplements different thematic explorations contingent on colonial medicine delineated above, including the biopolitical aspect of colonial governmentality, racial attributes of liberal colonial empire, attempts at the making of colonial selfhood by Indian reformers who sought modernization through vernacularization of medical knowledge, and operating of biopower, by viewing all these changes through the lens of gender. It seeks to address the function of liberalism in the realm of women's health, through the spread of educational and institutional changes, and reform of the zenana (women's quarters in upper-class Hindu and Muslim households), showing also how this led to the medicalization of women's bodies. Another broad theme explicated here is how gender was viewed and placed in the programme of reform and self-improvement through technologies of medicine adopted by colonial subjects. Sexual discourses, every-day practices in diet, household norms, and so forth, are analysed to evaluate dispensation of hygienic responsibilities. All this, undoubtedly, would eventually contribute towards enhancing and sharpening our understanding of what is colonial about colonial medicine by explicating the role played by gender in shaping it.

Scholars have pointed out that as the British 'extended their rule across the face of India during the late eighteenth and early nineteenth centuries, they had to confront the problem of how to govern this far-flung dependency, and, more importantly, how to justify this governance to themselves.'[24] To give shape to a coherent administrative policy, normative discourses were produced which tried to conceptualize, categorize, as well as essentialize the civilization of the East as the 'other' of the enlightened West. These discourses, however, were never static. They had complex and multiple dimensions, and passed through different trajectories.[25] Gender played a pivotal role in this discourse and so did science and medicine.

Gender figured overwhelmingly in the imperial civilizational discourses from an early period. As early as the 1750s, Robert Orme wrote: 'We see throughout India a race of men, whose make, physiognomy, and muscular strength convey ideas of an effeminacy which surprises when pursued through such numbers of the species, and when compared through the form of the European who is making observation.'[26] With the growth of the empire, the categories of gender came to increasingly influence notions of India's difference with the West and helped define ways to order the relations between the ruler and the ruled. Indian women were viewed as being degraded by Indian men—the markers for degradation being the zenana and the veil—and the British determined that they should become the rescuers and protectors of Indian women.

Medicine, on the other hand, came to occupy a dominant position among different scientific activities of European colonial powers in India since diseases of an unknown 'exotic' land had to be conceptualized and conquered in order to make commerce and colonization successful and enduring. As pointed out by scholars, the relationship between Western and non-Western medicines was variously shaped during different periods. From a relationship characterized by give and take between the Indian systems of medicine and Western medicine in the early seventeenth century, the British colonizers began to assume a sense of ideological and medical superiority in the aftermath of new scientific discoveries in the West.[27]

The colonial government, despite its inclination towards the use of effective Indian drugs, gradually propagated the colonial contention/dictum that Asian medical theories and practices were based on superstition and were inferior to Western science-based medicine. As pointed out by W. Ernst, 'science', as defined in Britain at the time, was the major yardstick for medical practice in the colony.[28] It had become linked with what Britain perceived to be its 'civilizing mission'. Ernst suggested, 'It was seen as infinitely superior, enlightened and rational, while India's many medical traditions and folk healing practices became increasingly denigrated as that which was inferior, traditional and backward, irrational and "other".'[29]

The view that had become increasingly widespread in the 1830s in India in the wake of the Anglicist/Orientalist debates was that few, if any, of the inhabitants of the globe are more completely under the control of superstition than the natives of Bengal. T.B. Macaulay, a staunch supporter and main protagonist of Anglicism, scornfully said that India held to 'medical doctrines which would disgrace an English farrier' and to an astronomy 'which would move laughter in girls at an English boarding school'.[30]

Condemnation of Indian Practices

Many commentators went so far as to claim that indigenous practitioners were shameless impostors who would not hesitate to use the most dangerous drugs and poisons on their patients.[31] From this viewpoint, eradication of indigenous practices would save the lives of people. This task could be best achieved through the dissemination of scientific medicine, and this became a part of the colonizers' civilizing mission. With this aim in view, the Calcutta Medical College (CMC) was established in 1835 as the first institution in India that exclusively taught scientific medicine.[32] Its predecessor, the Native Medical Institution (NMI), which opened in 1822, had offered courses in scientific medicine as well as in Ayurvedic and Unani medical systems. The language of instruction shifted from the vernacular at the NMI to English at the CMC.

When the CMC was instituted, its principal directed his attention primarily to the introduction of anatomy and practical dissection for three main reasons: (*a*) The absence of practical anatomy had been cited as one of the chief deficiencies of the NMI in the report that finally led to its abolition.[33] (*b*) The fact that dissections were not performed in contemporary India was also widely regarded as an aberration due to religious sentiments that directly contributed to the inferiority of indigenous medical knowledge. (*c*) Post-mortem anatomy was one of the most important aspects of scientific medicine, for it was perceived as the crucial way of coming to know the human body in its full depth.[34]

CMC established lying-in hospitals which admitted women, though women of higher classes and castes seldom showed eagerness to receive institutional care—at least till the latter half of the nineteenth century, when hospitals solely for women were established. The growth of study in human anatomy and physiology, nonetheless, had important implications for the study of the gendered body.

Themes

In order to throw light on this change, the first chapter deals with the growth of medical intervention through hospital medicine and traces the growth of lying-in hospitals attached to the CMC as well as other hospitals including the lock hospitals. It is shown how a space was created—albeit very small—for providing Western health care to women patients. Before the advent of hospital medicine, women were treated mostly by female practitioners of indigenous therapies who had commendable skills in this field. After the foundation of the Medical College in Calcutta in 1835, anatomical dissection was introduced in medical curricula and, consequently, an altogether different paradigm of knowledge emerged in the Indian context. Bedside medicine became less important than hospital medicine (when patients were transported to a 'noise-free' and detached medium of observation). Female patients (just as their male counterparts) were consequently subjected to an institutionally validated gaze.

The earliest institutions devoted to women's health were lock hospitals in different presidencies from around 1805, which were established for the confinement and treatment of prostitutes suspected of suffering from venereal diseases. Throughout the nineteenth century, venereal disease remained one of the most important causes of British troop admissions to hospitals in India. Lock hospitals were officially suppressed in 1833, only to be revived in 1868 under the Contagious Diseases Act (C.D. Act).[35]

Women officially registered as prostitutes under the C.D. Act of 1868 were compelled to attend the lock hospital for regular genital exams conducted by the presiding medical officer, and police were empowered to bring women who were suspected of prostitution to the lock hospital. If found to be diseased during the course of an examination, women could be incarcerated for treatment within the lock hospital until declared 'cured'.

Recent work has argued that the application of the Acts in the colonies distinguished itself from their operation within Britain because they reached much further into civil society and had primarily a punitive rather than a rehabilitative function. Most histories of the Indian Contagious Diseases Acts and their system of lock hospitals have situated them as part of a colonial rule of difference, in which the Acts were juridico-medical regimes that wrought a particularly pernicious form of social control upon an abject group.

It has been argued that the impact of the contagious diseases legislation in India introduced a new kind of bodily regulation in which the 'moral division between respectable and unrespectable women in India began to be detached from a sacred social hierarchy and became, instead, expressed through Western medical metaphors of health and disease'.[36]

In 1840, a large lying-in hospital was constructed on the grounds of the CMC through public subscriptions, followed by the opening of another hospital in 1852 where 116 beds out of a total of 350 accommodated women and children. Female patients belonging to different communities including Europeans, Eurasians, Mohammedans, and Hindus were treated in different medical establishments in Calcutta, among whom Hindus formed the largest single group. The discovery of chloroform in 1846–7 helped to popularize surgery to a certain extent. The number of female patients attending medical institutions remained very low and it was argued by both the British and the Indians that women were averse to treatment by male physicians. The supposed need to organize health care for reclusive Indian women made it easiest to find a moral consensus on women's medical education. Adas claims that the dissemination of scientific knowledge in general was one of the chief rationales for the extension of English education in India.[37]

The second chapter throws light on the origin and spread of medical education for women and the emergence of women medical practitioners. It portrays how the efforts of missionaries, government support, and the zeal of elite Indians for reform led to the opening up of medical education for women. The liberal phase of British administration in India saw an effort at social reform particularly aimed at women. The real objective was to bring Western enlightenment to the native Indian family by abolishing child marriage and sati, introducing remarriage of widows, and prohibiting other patriarchal customs that oppressed women. A vast body of the Anglo-Indian discursive writing that was produced in the second half of the nineteenth century focused critically on the condition of Indian women in the zenana. The zenana was considered to be a place of dirt, darkness, and disease.[38] The Christian missions' attempts at penetrating the zenana involved providing Westernized medical care to Indian women. In the 1850s, the Zenana Bible and Medical Missions started to send women missionaries and also lady doctors to women's quarters. In 1869, Dr Clara Swain, an American and the first fully qualified female medical missionary to get employment in India, was sent by the American Methodist Episcopal Mission to Bareilly. Fanny Butler, qualified from the London School of Medicine for Women, arrived in India in 1880 on behalf of the Church of England Zenana Missionary Society.[39]

It has been pointed out that before long, 'missions on both sides of the Atlantic began to champion the ability of women to apply the "double cure"': 'Healing the body while they healed the spirit'.[40] The opening up of medical education for female students in Europe and America, combined with the relatively fewer employment opportunities for women doctors than male medical practitioners there, facilitated the entry of Western women doctors to India. Madras Medical College provided medical education for women since 1875. In Bengal, the majority members of the Council of the CMC opposed the idea that women should be given medical training. According to them, women would better serve as nurses or midwives. Brahmo reformers were vocal about the need for opening up medical education to women, and government officials also favoured this. In the support for women's admission into medical colleges and schools, the colonial rulers saw the chance to boost their claim to commitment towards 'public good'. Qualified female physicians gained employment in zenana hospitals opened by the Dufferin Fund or the National Association for Supplying Female Medical Aid to the Women of India, which was organized in 1885 at the personal initiative of Queen Victoria. The queen was informed by Mary Scharlieb (wife of an English barrister, she received midwifery training in Madras and later became a London gynaecologist) and Elizabeth Bielby (missionary doctor at Lahore) about the lack of medical care for Indian women, following which the monarch asked Lady Harriot Dufferin, the new vicereine, to investigate about the scope of providing medical help to Indian women. On her initiative, the Fund was established in August 1885 with three aims: (*a*) to provide medical teaching and training to women; (*b*) to organize medical relief; and (*c*) to make the services of female nurses and midwives available in hospitals and private houses.[41]

Zenana hospitals instituted by the Fund, however, were not above criticism for practising racial discrimination appointing white-skinned doctors in preference to experienced and qualified Indian doctors.

Long before the organization of female medical care by branches of the Dufferin Fund, maternal care and infant care were sought to be reformed by the institutionalization of midwifery training. In Bengal (as in other parts of India), childbirth, which was regarded as a polluted task, was attended by indigenous *dhais* or traditional birth attendants who were mostly members of the lower castes in the hierarchy of the Hindu society, or were poor Muslim women. In the course of the nineteenth century, they became the symbols of 'superstition and dogged resistance to change'.[42]

In fact, throughout the nineteenth century, traditional Indian birthing practices were under the scrutiny of both Bengali and British reformers. Missionaries and British doctors believed that the unscientific practices promoted by the midwives, or birth attendants, or dhais (as midwives were colloquially known), and unhygienic condition of the *anturghar* or *sutikagriha* (where birthing took place), were the main causes of the appallingly high rates of maternal mortality in India.

The medicalization of childbirth became part of distinct, professionalized fields of medical expertise and practice. In Bengal, an indigenous practitioner of medicine was the first to draw attention to the need to train traditional birth attendants. In the early half of the nineteenth century, the Fever Hospital Committee was formed by Governor General Auckland in 1835. It consulted evidence gathered from laypersons as well as medical men—both Europeans and Indians—on subjects such as Calcutta's drainage system, water supply, tanks, ventilation, roads, and even native habits that might pose danger to health. Responding to the Fever Hospital Committee's queries on native life, Madhusudan Gupta had testified on the poor state of women's health. He pointed out that as a result of the primitive management of childbirth, three to four women of twenty died of fever or tetanus.[43] In his opinion, midwifery training should be imparted to improve the system of birth management.

In Bengal, institutionalized training programmes for midwives were finally introduced in the 1870s. One obvious limitation of these programmes was that because of the necessity of some degree of knowledge of English and regular attendance, there were very few respondents from among the economically impoverished section of the dhais belonging to lower castes. Sometimes, however, training in these programmes opened up avenues of lucrative employment for those belonging to urban and semi-urban groups.

Attempts to medicalize childbirth cannot be understood as simply an effect of improved clinical outcomes, rather we must also investigate this history in terms of how new practices were imbued with positive social, political, and cultural values. For the colonized people, modernization of traditional midwifery was part of the self-perceptions and desire for self-improvement and formulation of middle-class identity. For the upper castes, sanitized cleanliness became an ideology for asserting its own identity, as it worked in tandem with notions of caste purity and pollution. The emphasis on unsanitary practices of the traditional birth attendants made them more and more marginalized in the emerging discourse on science and modernity.

Chapter 3 portrays how reproductive health was sought to be modernized by different means. Apart from the institutionalization of midwifery training, another important method was to spread new knowledge of prenatal and postnatal care through guidebooks and essays addressed to expectant mothers. Jadunath Mukhopadhyaya, Licentiate in Medicine and Surgery (LMS) of CMC, wrote *Dhatrisiksha ebong Prasutisiksha: A Guide to Native Midwives & Mothers* in two volumes (first published in 1867). *Saral Dhatrisiksha* written by Sundarimohan Das (M.B., Professor of Midwifery of Physician and Surgeon College) was published in B.S. 1308 (1901). These manuals were written in simple and homely Bengali. In 1867, the *Bama bodhini patrika* published a series of detailed and informative articles on midwifery, covering pregnancy, its symptoms and treatment, and delivery. Manuals on household hints and collections of essays for the purpose of female education also contained sections on midwifery. The nineteenth century also saw the publication of a large number of writings of physicians as well as social reformers, which addressed the subject of the degeneration of health of Bengalis, including discussions on the causes and remedies of this situation.

Apart from environmental factors, social customs, and bodily practices like child marriage, harmful sexual behaviours, and so on were blamed for making the physique weak and fragile. Women were often portrayed as victims as well as agents of degeneration. As biological reproducers of the race, mothers and good wives were required to give birth to and raise healthy children who would become the representatives of a strong, masculine nation. Health advice mostly intended for women readers formed part of the new discourse of domesticity, shaped partly by the need to respond to the colonial critique of Indian norms of family life (internalized by the colonized middle class) and by the necessity to adjust to colonial rule. This new discourse was rooted in the felt need to formulate an indigenous ideal of modernity which would be imbued by the precepts of Western science and medicine and was perceived to be the foundation of the restructuring of the nation.

The fourth chapter throws light on multiple aspects of these discussions and their significance for women. Many of these new discourses on sexuality and domestic practices focused on the remodelling of women's role as health-conscious good wives and mothers. Many Bengali periodicals pointed out that social customs like child marriages, as well as harmful practices like masturbation and nocturnal pollution, indiscriminate coital indulgence, and even excessive sexual intercourse with one's own husband might harm a woman's health, leading to maternal mortality or the birth of sick babies.

Medical and quasi-medical literature of this period included guidelines for an ideal housewife for proper home management, scientific nurturing of children, regulation of dietary habits, creation of hygienic environment, and so forth. Women were expected to know a bit of all available forms of treatment, including folk medicine, allopathy, homeopathy, *kabiraji* (therapeutic practices followed by a *kabiraj* or practitioner of Ayurvedic medicine), and *hakimi* (therapeutic practices followed by practitioners of Unani medicine). Parents, particularly mothers, were advised to educate themselves to be able to understand and execute the medical experts' instructions. This in a way augmented women's power. Biographical evidence shows that some women did try to follow the advice given in the manuals.

It is interesting to note how the new discourses on sexuality and domesticity, of which health advice formed an inseparable and important component, aimed at reformulating the private domain of the nation coincided with debates and demands of marriage reforms. Since the second half of the nineteenth century, social reformers invoked physiological issues in debates on raising the age of marriage. During the child marriage controversies of the 1860s and 1870s, ultimately resulting in the Native Marriage Act of 1872, Keshab Chandra Sen, the leader of the Sadharan Brahmo Samaj, solicited the opinions of doctors practising in Bengal on the effect of different influences—including climate and other factors—on tropical bodies, in a quest for determining what should be the earliest age of marriage from the point of view of the well-being of the mother, the child, and society.

It was the earliest example of an appeal to physiology for rationalizing social reform. During the Age of Consent controversy in the 1890s following the death of Phulmoni Dasi, eleven, who died of injuries inflicted on her wedding night by her husband Hari Mohan Maiti, thirty-seven, the discussions of both the supporters of increasing the age of consent from ten to twelve, as well as those of the orthodox opposition, were rendered in the language of physiology and medicine.

In the twentieth century, the Marriage Reform Act or Sarda Act of 1929 (like the Act of 1891) was also partly debated on medical grounds. There was comparatively less opposition to the matter of raising the age of permissible sexual intercourse in marriage, and this can be explained at least partially by the entry of women's organizations into the public sphere. This and other changes of the early twentieth century related to women's health, form the subject matter of the fifth chapter. Chapter 5 throws light on the changing nature of health care practices in the late colonial era, which put emphasis on disseminating and popularizing health education among women through different agencies against the background of late colonial political and socio-economic situation. There was growth of voluntary associations devoted to maternal as well as child health care. The government offered financial help to the local bodies and voluntary organizations for the establishment and maintenance of maternity and child welfare centres, and for the organization of maternity services.

Following the example of the Dufferin Fund, different voluntary organizations set up by imperial women like the Lady Reading Fund and the Lady Chelmsford Fund became involved in organizing health care activities for women and children. Organization of baby shows and welfare exhibitions, sale of medical literature, public health education, and child welfare centres were patterned on the Western model, which would supposedly provide better health and longer lifespan for women and children.

The first half of the twentieth century also experienced heightened public interest and veritable discourses on body and sexuality against the background of intensification of the nationalist struggle and vociferous criticism of Indian social practices by the imperialists. Maternal and child welfare, demographic reform, national strength—regarded as features of modern public health sensibilities—linked the welfare of the individual body to the emergence of a strong nation.

Under the influence of eugenics societies, the health of each nation became associated with increasing the physical strength and purity of the 'race', scientifically brought up by hygienically enlightened mothers. Women physicians as well as nationalist reformers and social and political organizations sought to contribute to eugenic reforms through their support of birth control. Birth control and eugenics, supported by international efforts and initiatives of private Indians, became objects of immense attention.[44]

Since 1919, health came under the purview of the provincial government. Public health records around the end of the 1930s drew attention to the simultaneous deterioration in respect of both births and death rates. The rate of stillbirths was steadily rising as also the death rate from maternal causes. Chapter 6 draws attention to the growth of public health care administration and its impact on women's health, finally ending with an account of the devastating result of the famine of 1943–4. During the famine, women died in large numbers not only due to famine-induced epidemics, but also because they suffered abandonment and destitution, leading to the adoption of survival strategies which affected health status. The famine exposed how poor health status, inefficiency of public health administration, dietary deficiency among Indians, particularly among women and children, and so on, made them extremely vulnerable to starvation-induced deaths, further lowering the health status of women.

Undoubtedly, not every possible aspect related to women and medicine in colonial Bengal can be covered in this book. Paucity or inaccessibility of primary data has sometimes hindered deeper engagement with various issues. I wish to stress that the shape of any work of history is determined by the nature of the available material. It is on the foundation of such material that the structure of this work is built.

Some of the essential and significant features related to women's health care in colonial India that have been addressed here would help us understand how far and in what ways gender and medicine worked as integral parts of colonialism and in the unfolding of the ideas of India's modernity, which over the years became part of Indians' selfhood. Here two approaches are combined to study different aspects related to women and medicine—one may be called the 'women in medicine' approach which tries to focus on women in medical policy and practice, implying a study of how far they were integrated into changes which occurred in the field of medicine and health care; the other follows what may be termed as the 'gender and medicine' approach to explore how new discursive domains of medical knowledge helped formulate certain stereotypes based on the spread of gynaecological knowledge through the growth of different institutions as well as new regimes of knowledge as corollary to biomedicine. On the whole, these analyses will no doubt help to generate new questions and issues, which one might hope will be taken up in future by new researchers in the field.

Notes and References

1. Some of the important works focusing on gender and colonialism/imperialism are: Nupur Chaudhuri and Margaret Strobel, eds, *Western Women and Imperialism: Complicity and Resistance* (Bloomington: Indiana University Press, 1992); Antoinette Burton, *Burdens of History: British Feminists, Indian Women and Imperial Culture, 1865–1915* (Chapel Hill, London: University of North Carolina, 1994); Clare Midgeley, ed., *Gender and Imperialism* (Manchester: Manchester University Press, 1998); Mary Procida, *Married to the Empire: Gender, Politics and Imperialism in India, 1883–1947* (Manchester and New York: Manchester University Press, 2002); Philippa Levine, ed., *Gender and Empire* (Oxford: Oxford University Press, 2004).

2. Some of the recent writings in the field are as follows: Arnold P. Kaminsky, 'Morality Legislation and British Troops in Late Nineteenth-Century India', *Military Affairs*, 43 (1979): 78–83; Kenneth Ballhatchet, *Race, Sex and Class*

under the Raj: Imperial Attitudes, and Policies and Their Critics, 1793–1905 (London: Weidenfeld and Nicolson, 1980); Barbara Ramusack, 'Embattled Advocates: The Debate over Birth Control in India, 1920–1940', *Journal of Women's History* 1, no. 2 (1989): 34–74; P. Jeffrey, R. Jeffrey, and A. Lyon, *Labour Pains and Labour Power: Women and Childbearing in India* (London: Zed Books, 1989); Antoinette Burton, 'The White Woman's Burden: British Feminists and the 'Indian Woman', 1865–1915', in N. Chaudhuri and Strobel, *Western Women and Imperialism* (1992), pp. 137–57; Barbara Ramusack, 'Cultural Missionaries, Maternal Imperialists: Feminist Allies: British Women Activists in India, 1865–1945', in N. Chaudhuri and Strobel, *Western Women and Imperialism* (1992), pp. 119–36; Dagmar Engels, 'The Politics of Childbirth: British and Bengali Women in Contest, 1890–1930', in *Society and Ideology: Essays in South Asian History*, edited by Peter Robb (New Delhi: Oxford University Press, 1993), pp. 222–46; David Arnold, 'Sexually Transmitted Diseases in Nineteenth- and Twentieth-Century India', *Genitourinary Medicine* 69 (1993): 3–8; Geraldine Forbes, 'Managing Midwifery in India', in *Contesting Colonial Hegemony: State and Society in Africa and India*, edited by Dagmar Engels and Shula Marks (London: British Academic Press, 1994), pp. 152–72; Maneesha Lal, 'The Politics of Gender and Medicine in Colonial India: The Countess of Dufferin's Fund, 1885–1888', *Bulletin of the History of Medicine* 68, no. 1 (1994): 29–66; Philippa Levine, 'Venereal Disease, Prostitution, and the Politics of Empire: The Case of British India', *Journal of the History of Sexuality* 4 (1994): 579–602; Judy Whitehead, 'Bodies Clean and Unclean: Prostitution, Sanitary Legislation and Respectable Femininity in Colonial North India', *Gender and History* 7, no. 1 (1995): 41–63; Antoinette Burton, 'Contesting the Zenana: The Mission to Make "Lady Doctors for India", 1874–1885', *Journal of British Studies* 35, no. 3 (1996): 368–97; Supriya Guha, 'The Unwanted Pregnancy in Colonial Bengal', *Indian Economic and Social History Review* 33 no. 4 (1996): 403–35; Waltraud Ernst, 'European Madness and Gender in Nineteenth Century British India', *Social History Medicine* 9, no. 3 (1996): 357–82; S. Anandhi, 'Reproductive Bodies and Regulated Sexuality: Birth Control Debates in Early Twentieth Century Tamilnadu', in *A Question of Silence? The Sexual Economics of Modern India*, edited by Mary E. John and Janaki Nair (New Delhi: Kali for Women, 1998), pp. 139–66; Geraldine Forbes, 'Introduction to Memoirs', in *The Memoirs of Dr. Haimabati Sen: From Child Widow to Lady Doctor*, edited by Geraldine Forbes and Tapan Raychaudhuri (New Delhi: Roli Books, 2000), pp. 152–72; Maina Chawla Singh, *Gender, Religion and 'Heathen Lands': American Missionary Women in South Asia (1860–1940s)* (New York: Garland, 2000); Sarah Hodges, ed., *Reproductive Health in India: History, Politics and Controversies* (New Delhi: Orient Longman, 2000); Anshu Malhotra, 'Of Dais and Midwives, "Middle Class" Interventions in the Management of Women's Reproductive Health; A Study from Colonial Punjab', *Indian Journal of Gender Studies* 10, no. 2 (2003): 229–59; Philippa Levine, *Prostitution, Race and Polities Policing Venereal Disease in the British Empire* (London: Routledge, 2003); Charu Gupta, 'Procreation and Pleasure: Writings of a Woman Ayurvedic Practitioner in Colonial North India', *Studies in History* 21, no. 1 (2005): 17–44; Indrani Sen, 'The Memsahib's "Madness": The European Woman's Mental Health in Late Nineteenth Century India', *Social Scientist* 33, nos 5–6 (2005): 26–48; Maina Chawla Singh, 'Gender, Medicine and Empire: Early Initiatives in Institution Building and Professionalisation (1890s–1940s),' in *Exploring Gender Equations: Colonial and Post Colonial India*, edited by Shakti Kak and Biswamoy Pati (New Delhi: Nehru Memorial Museum and Library, 2005), pp. 93–115; Samikhsha Sehrawat, 'The Foundation of the Lady Hardinge Medical College and Hospital for Women at Delhi: Issues in Women's Medical Education and Imperial Governance' (2005), in Kak and Pati, *Exploring Gender Equations*, pp. 117–46; Sean Lang, 'Drop the Demon Dai: Maternal Mortality and the State in Colonial Madras, 1840–1875', *Social History of Medicine* 18, no. 3 (2005): 357–78; Waltraud Ernst, 'Feminising Madness—Feminising the Orient: Madness, Gender and Colonialism in British India, 1860–1940', in Kak and Pati, *Exploring Gender Equations* (2005), pp. 57–91; Rosemary Fitzgerald, '"Making and Moulding the Nursing of the Indian Empire", Recasting Nurses in Colonial India', in *Gender and the Colonial Experience in South Asia*, edited by Avril A. Powell and Siobhan Lambert Hurley (New Delhi: Oxford University Press, 2006); Samita Sen and Anirban Das, 'A History of the Calcutta Medical College and Hospital, 1835–1936', in *Science and Modern India: An Institutional History, c. 1784–1947* edited by Uma Das Gupta, *Project of History of Science, Philosophy and Culture in Indian Civilization*, vol. 15, Part 4 (2010), pp. 477–522; Mridula Ramanna, *Health Care in Bombay Presidency, 1896–1930* (New Delhi: Primus Books, 2012); Samiksha Sehrawat, *Colonial Medical Care in North India: Gender, State, and Society, c. 1840–1920* (New Delhi: Oxford University Press, 2013); Debjani Das, *Houses of Madness: Insanity and Asylums of Bengal in Nineteenth-Century India* (New Delhi: Oxford University Press, 2015).

3. David Arnold, for example, points out that in the early nineteenth century, 'in an essentially male-oriented and male-operated system of medicine, women appeared only as adjuncts and appendages to the health of men.' He also writes: 'The primary areas of state medicine in the first half of the nineteenth century—the army, the jails, even the hospitals—were primarily male domains in which women played little part.' See David Arnold, *Colonizing the Body: State Medicine and Epidemic Disease in Nineteenth-Century India* (New Delhi: Oxford University Press, 1993), p. 254.

4. See Daniel R. Headrick, *The Tools of Empire: Technology and European Imperialism in the Nineteenth Century* (New York: Oxford University Press, 1981); Philip D. Curtin, *The Image of Africa: British Ideas and Action, 1780–1850* (Madison: University of Wisconsin Press, 1964); Philip D. Curtin, *Death by Migration: Europe's Encounter with the Tropical World in the Nineteenth Century* (Cambridge: Cambridge University Press, 1989).

5. Arnold, *Colonizing the Body*, p. 8.

6. Waltraud Ernst, 'Beyond East and West: From the History of Colonial Medicine to a Social History of Medicine(s) in South Asia', *Social History of Medicine* 20, no. 3 (13 November 2007): 505–24. Also cited in Prajit Bihari Mukharji, *Nationalizing the Body: The Medical Market, Print and Daktari Medicine* (London: Anthem Press, 2009), p. 8n32.

7. Waltraud Ernst, *Mad Tales from the Raj: European Insane in British India* (London: Routledge, 1991). Also cited in Mukharji, *Nationalizing the Body*, p. 17n84.

8. Arnold, *Colonizing the Body*, p. 9.

9. Arnold, *Colonizing the Body*, p. 9.

10. Mark Harrison, *Public Health in British India: Anglo–Indian Preventive Medicine 1859–1914* (New Delhi: Cambridge University Press, Foundation Books, 1994).

11. Radhika Ramasubban, 'Public Health and Medical Research in India: Their Origins under the Impact of British Colonial Policy', *SAREC Report* (Stockholm, 1982); Radhika Ramasubban, 'Imperial Health in British India, 1857–1900', in *Disease, Medicine and Empire: Perspectives on Western Medicine and the Experience of European Expansion*, edited by Roy Macleod and Milton Lewis (London: Routledge, 1988), pp. 38–60.

12. See Mark Harrison, 'Medicine and Orientalism: Perspectives on Europe's Encounter with Indian Medical Systems', in *Health, Medicine and Empire: Perspectives on Colonial India*, edited by Biswamoy Pati and Mark Harrison (New Delhi: Orient Longman, 2001), pp. 37–87.

13. Ishita Pande, *Medicine, Race and Liberalism in British Bengal: Symptoms of Empire* (London and New York: Routledge, 2010), p. 7; Partha Chatterjee, *The Nation and Its Fragments: Colonial and Postcolonial Histories* (New Delhi: Oxford University Press, 1992), p. 14.

14. See Ann Laura Stoler, *Race and the Education of Desire: Foucault's 'History of Sexuality' and the Colonial Order of Things* (Durham: Duke University Press, 1995).

15. Gyan Prakash, *Another Reason: Science and the Imagination of Modern India* (New Delhi: Oxford University Press, 2000), p. 127.

16. Pande, *Medicine, Race and Liberalism*, p. 6. Throughout this book, the word 'native' has been used as in official records of the time and as an opposite for the category 'European'.

17. Pande, *Medicine, Race and Liberalism*, p. 7.

18. David Arnold, *The Tropics and the Traveling Gaze: India, Landscape, and Science, 1800–1856* (Seattle: University of Washington Press, 2006).

19. Pande, *Medicine, Race and Liberalism*, p. 15.

20. Mukharji, *Nationalizing the Body*, p. 29.

21. Megan Vaughan, *Curing Their Ills: Colonial Power and African Illness* (Stanford: Stanford University Press, 1991), p. 25, cited in Mukharji, *Nationalizing the Body*, p. 10n46.

22. Sander L. Gilman, 'The Hottentot and the Prostitute: Towards an Iconography of Female Sexuality', in *Difference and Pathology: Stereotypes of Sexuality, Race, and Madness*, edited by Sander L. Gilman (Ithaca: Cornell University Press, 1985), p. 83.

23. Shula Marks, 'What Is Colonial about Colonial Medicine? And What Has Happened to Imperialism and Health?' *Social History of Medicine* 10 (1997): 210. Also cited in Pande, *Medicine, Race and Liberalism*, p. 10n48. Shula Marks, 'What Is Colonial about Colonial Medicine? And What Has Happened to Imperialism and Health?' *Social History of Medicine* 10 (1997): 210. Also cited in Pande, *Medicine, Race and Liberalism*, p. 10n48.

24. Thomas R. Metcalf, *The New Cambridge History of India*, vol. 3, part 4, *Ideologies of the Raj* (New Delhi: Foundation Books, 1995), p. 1.

25. Edward Said has suggested that neither imperialism nor colonialism is a simple act of accumulation. Both are supported and perhaps even impelled by impressive ideological formations that include notions that certain territories and people require and beseech domination, as well as forms of knowledge affiliated with domination. The vocabulary of the classic nineteenth-century imperial culture is plentiful with such words and concepts as 'inferior' or 'subject races', 'subordinate peoples', 'dependency', 'expansion', and 'authority'. (Edward W. Said, *Culture and Imperialism* [New York: Vintage Books, 1994], p. 9.)

26. Robert Orme, *Government and the People of Indostan*, part 1 (London, 1753; reprinted in Lucknow, 1971), pp. 42–3. Cited in Metcalf, *The New Cambridge History*, p. 93.

27. See Harrison, 'Medicine and Orientalism', pp. 37–87.

28. Waltraud Ernst, 'Colonial Psychiatry, Magic and Religion: The Case of Mesmerism in British India', *History of Psychiatry* 15, no. 1 (2004): 57–71.

29. Ernst, 'Colonial Psychiatry, Magic and Religion': 61.

30. W.T. DeBary, *Sources of Indian Tradition* (New York: Columbia University Press, 1968).

31. James Ranald Martin, *Notes on the Medical Topography of Calcutta* (Calcutta, 1837); C.E. Trevelyan, *Education of the People of India* (1838). Quoted

in *Higher Education in Bengal under British Rule*, by Jajneswar Ghosh (Calcutta: Book Company, 1926), p. 108.

32. For the development of medical education in colonial Bengal, see Om Prakash Jaggi, 'Advent of English Medical Education in India', in *Science, Philosophy and Culture: Multidisciplinary Explorations*, part I, edited by B.D. Chattopadhyaya and Ravinder Kumar (New Delhi: PHISPC, 1996), pp. 427–64; and Anil Kumar, *Medicine and the Raj: British Medical Policy in India*, 1835–1911 (New Delhi: SAGE Publications, 1998), pp. 19–36. On university education in general, see J.F. Hilliker, 'The Creation of a Middle Class as a Goal of Educational Policy in Bengal, 1833–1854', in *Indian Society and the Beginnings of Modernisation, c. 1830–1850*, edited by Cyril Philips and Mary Wainwright (London: University of London School of Oriental and African Studies, 1976), pp. 31–43; and Dagmar Engels, 'Modes of Knowledge, Modes of Power: Universities in Nineteenth-Century India', in *Contesting Colonial Hegemony: State and Society in Africa and India*, edited by Dagmar Engels and Shula Marks (London: British Academic Press, 1994), pp. 87–109. For studies on the intellectual milieu of nineteenth-century Bengal, see especially Tapan Raychaudhuri, *Europe Reconsidered: Perceptions of the West in Nineteenth-Century Bengal* (New Delhi: Oxford University Press, 1988) and his 'The Pursuit of Reason in Nineteenth-Century Bengal', in his *Perceptions, Emotions, Sensibilities: Essays on India's Colonial and Post-Colonial Experiences* (New Delhi: Oxford University Press, 1999), pp. 49–65. See also Sibnarayan Ray, *Bengal Renaissance: The First Phase* (Calcutta: Minerva Associates, 2000), pp. 49–67, 90–114.

33. 'Report of the Native Medical Institution Committee, with the Measures Adopted Consequent Thereon', *Board's Collections*, F/4/1527, 1835–36, vol. 1527 (London: Oriental and India Office Collections, British Library), p. 107. Cited in Christian Hochmuth, 'Patterns of Medical Culture in Colonial Bengal, 1835–1880', *Bulletin of the History of Medicine* 80 (2006): 39–72. A summary of the report can be found in Zhaleh Khaleeli, 'Harmony or Hegemony? The Rise and Fall of the Native Medical Institution, Calcutta; 1822–35', *South Asia Research* 21 (2001): 77–104, on 88–93.

34. This idea actually derives from the Renaissance tradition of human dissection. See, for example, Jonathan Sawday, *The Body Emblazoned: Dissection and the Human Body in Renaissance Culture* (London: Routledge, 1995).

35. For a discussion regarding lock hospitals, venereal diseases, the Contagious Diseases Acts, and other related topics, see Kaminsky, 'Morality Legislation and British Troops in Late Nineteenth-Century India' (1979): 78–83; Ballhatchet, *Race, Sex and Class under the Raj* (1980); Ratnabali Chatterjee, 'The Indian Prostitute as a Colonial Subject, Bengal 1864–1883',

Canadian Woman Studies/Les Cahiers de la Femme 13, no. 1 (1992): 51–5; Arnold, 'Sexually Transmitted Diseases in Nineteenth- and Twentieth-Century India' (1993): 3–8; M. Sundara Raj, *Prostitution in Madras, A Study in Historical Perspective* (New Delhi: Konark Publications Pvt. Ltd, 1993); Miles Ogborn, 'Law and Discipline in Nineteenth Century English State Formation: The Contagious Diseases Acts of 1864, 1866, and 1869', *Journal of Historical Sociology* 6, no. 1 (1993): 28–55; Sumanta Banerjee, 'The "Beshya" and the "Babu": Prostitute and Her Clientele in 19th Century Bengal', *Economic and Political Weekly* 28, no. 45 (1993): 2461–72; Burton, *Burdens of History* (1994); Levine, 'Venereal Disease, Prostitution, and the Politics of Empire' (1994): 579–60; Whitehead, 'Bodies Clean and Unclean' (1995): 41–63; Philippa Levine, 'Rereading the 1890s: Venereal Disease as "Constitutional Crisis" in Britain and British India', *Journal of Asian Studies* 55, no. 3 (August 1996): 585–612; Douglas M. Peers, 'Soldiers, Surgeons and the Campaigns to Combat Sexually Transmitted Diseases in Colonial India, 1805–1860', *Medical History* 42, no. 2 (April 1998): 137–60; Mridula Ramanna, 'Control and Resistance: The Working of the Contagious Diseases Acts in Bombay City', *Economic and Political Weekly* 35, no. 17 (22 April 2000): 1470–6; Sabyasachi R. Mishra, 'An Empire "De-Masculinized": The British Colonial State and the Problem of Syphilis in Nineteenth-Century India', in *Disease and Medicine in India: A Historical Overview*, edited by Deepak Kumar (New Delhi: Tulika, 2001), pp. 166–79; Stephen Legg, 'Governing Prostitution in Colonial Delhi: From Cantonment Regulations to International Hygiene (1864–1939)', *Social History* 34, no. 4 (November 2009): 447–67; Sujata Mukherjee, 'Imperialism, Medicine and Women's Health in Nineteenth Century India', in *Science and Society in India, c. 1750–2000*, edited by Arun Bandopadhyay (New Delhi: Manohar, 2010), pp. 95–120.

36. Whitehead, 'Bodies Clean and Unclean': 41, cited in David Arnold, *The New Cambridge History of India*, vol. 3, part 5, *Science, Technology and Medicine in Colonial India* (Cambridge: Cambridge University Press, 2002), p. 90.

37. Michael Adas, 'Scientific Standards and Colonial Education in British India and French Senegal', in *Science, Medicine and Cultural Imperialism*, edited by Teresa Meade and Mark Walker (Basingstoke: Macmillan, 1991), pp. 4–35, on p. 20.

38. Janaki Nair, 'Uncovering the Zenana: Visions of Indian Womanhood in Englishwomen's Writings, 1813–1940', *Journal of Women's History* 2, no. 11 (Spring 1990): 8–34.

39. Arnold, *The New Cambridge History of India*, vol. 3, part 5, *Science, Technology and Medicine in Colonial India*, p. 87.

40. Geraldine Forbes, 'Colonial Imperatives and Women's Emancipation: Western Medical Education for Indian Women in Nineteenth Century Bengal',

Modern Historical Studies 2 (2001), Journal of the Department of History, Rabindra Bharati University: 83–102.

41. On the Fund's early activities, see Lal, 'The Countess of Dufferin's Fund, 1885–1888'.

42. Forbes, 'Managing Midwifery in India', p. 171.

43. Fever Hospital Committee, *Abridgement of the Report of the Committee Appointed by the Right Honorable the Governor of Bengal for the Establishment of a Fever Hospital and for Inquiring into Local Management and Taxation in Calcutta* (Calcutta: 1840), pp. 62–3.

44. Ramusack, 'Embattled Advocates': 34–64; Anandhi, 'Reproductive Bodies and Regulated Sexuality', pp. 139–66; Mausumi Manna, 'Approach towards Birth Control: Indian Women in the Early Twentieth Century', *IESHR* 35, no. 1 (1998): 35–51; Sanjam Ahluwalia, *Reproductive Restraints: Birth Control in India 1877–1947* (New Delhi: Permanent Black, 2008).

1 *Western Medicine, Hospitals, and Female Health in Nineteenth-Century Bengal*

CHRONIC RHEUMATISM
June 15, 1847. Munnoojohn, a peasant woman, aged 40, residing in Calcutta, has been suffering from chronic rheumatism for a year, with pain, weakness and partial loss of feeling of both legs extending up to the waist. It is attended with a peculiar pricking sensation of the legs, and the left one is much wasted, she can walk a little with the assistance of a staff, but limps much at the time, she cannot raise herself up from sitting posture, even with the help of a stick.

NEURALGIA
July 4, 1847. Bebee Punnah, a peasant woman, aged 50, residing at Taltullah, in Calcutta, has been tormented for three months with neuralgic pains shooting from the neck down to the waist, both before and behind, and increasingly much at night, preventing her sleep, the least movement increases her suffering.

The two extracts at the beginning of this chapter are taken from *Record of Cases Treated in the Mesmeric Hospital* during 1847.[1] The Mesmeric Hospital, which was commonly known among the lower classes of the Indian population as the *house of magic* or *jadoo* hospital, seemed to be visited more frequently by Indians unlike some other colonial medical institutions set up by the British.[2] Its founder was Dr James Esdaile, the son of a Scottish clergyman and brother of the Reverend David Esdaile of Forfar, who came to Calcutta after completing his medical training at the University of Edinburgh in 1830 to work as a surgeon. He became the Civil Surgeon in Hoogli and acted as principal of the Hoogli College from 1839 to 1847. Esdaile began his experiments in mesmerism in 1845 and performed his first operation in April 1845. It was followed by seventy-three more operations within the next eight months. These included amputations and also 'removal of Tumours on patients rendered unconscious by mesmerism.'[3] After his success in mesmerism, the government allotted a room in the Calcutta Native Hospital, which would accommodate ten patients, for operations under mesmerism. A committee of seven members was also appointed to report on Esdaile's experiments. Following the favourable report submitted by the committee, a mesmeric hospital was established in Mott's Lane in Calcutta in November 1846. Here 'cases of all kinds were admitted and operated on, under the mesmeric influence, by Esdaile.'[4]

Sometimes treatment was slow and the result could be delayed. It was recorded that the two peasant women mentioned earlier were treated and cured by mesmerism, but in the case of Munnoojohn, after the treatment of mesmerizing her daily for an hour and half started, for some days there was an aggravation of the symptoms, followed by a severe fever. By 20 July, the fever left her and the pain and swelling of the shoulders were gone. She could move her arms freely and the pricking of the limbs was much reduced. Gradually the pain disappeared. Within another week, she started walking. On 13 August 1847, she said that she had become well and wanted to go home, and was subsequently discharged.

Bebee Punnah, the patient suffering from neuralgia, was mesmerized for an hour daily and on the very first day she felt relief of the pain in her waist and back. By 14 August 1847, she could bend her neck freely like any other person and perceived no pain. She could even walk without any inconvenience. As her situation improved and her pain was gone, she was released from the hospital.

The application of ether (1846) and chloroform (1847) made painless surgery not only possible, but also available at much less cost than mesmo-surgery since medical assistants had to spend less time on pre-operative mesmeric sessions.[5] Thus, the major reason to lend support to Esdaile's approach disappeared around this time. After the closing of the mesmeric hospital, Esdaile was appointed superintendent of the Sukea Street Dispensary and continued to practise mesmerism till he left India in June 1851.[6]

Long before the foundation of the Mesmeric Hospital, Calcutta witnessed the establishment of a number of hospitals and lunatic asylums, starting with the General Hospital, founded in 1707 for the treatment of East India Company's soldiers and sailors. The efficiency of treatment, however, remained doubtful. Captain Alexander Hamilton, a sailor, who stayed there in 1708 remarked: 'The Company has a pretty good hospital at Calcutta, where many go in to undergo the penance of physic, but few come out to give an account of its operation.'[7] The Presidency General Hospital was started in 1768 to accommodate European patients. In 1787, the government took the initiative to establish the Dum Dum Hospital chiefly for vaccine inoculation among soldiers and their families. Asylums for Indian lunatics were also established quite early. The court of directors of the East India Company decreed in 1802 that lunatic asylums for the reception of both criminal and freely wandering insane Indians ought to be established in Bengal. By 1820, a number of lunatic asylums for the exclusive reception of Indians (and of the lowest strata of Eurasians) had been established. In the Bengal Presidency provisions for the care of mad persons were made in Calcutta, Bareilly, Benares, Dhaka, Murshidabad, and Patna. One aspect of asylum management that was criticized was the inadequate segregation of patients in general and the improper mixing of men and women in particular. It was suggested that due attention be paid to the separation. Official records of the 1850s designated many inmates as 'paupers', consisting of 'nearly 2/3 of the admissions of religious mendicants, Outcastes and prostitutes'.[8]

A police hospital was set up in Calcutta around 1789, which received 'poor wretches...those who are perfectly destitute and found lying about in the streets'.[9] Apparently 'the establishment of an Institution for the relief of Natives suffering from accidents and sickness was proposed to the community in the year 1792'.[10] Its purpose was primarily to give medicines to the injured in accidents. There was an opinion that hospitals should be opened to serve the productive section, not only beggars and the destitute. Testimonies of European doctors attached to different hospitals show that momentum gathered to regulate the productive section of the Indian population. There was a demand for a new hospital not for 'beggars and destitute, but for a better class, such as the servants of the Baboos and other wealthy natives, also for Musselmen and Hindoos, and the servants of European families in general'.[11] An urge was felt to set up a new 'Fever' hospital to deal with the outbreak of epidemics. The Fever Hospital Committee commissioned by Lord Auckland in 1835 consisted of doctors and administrators who gathered evidence from doctors and laypersons, and pored over plans for Calcutta's improvement. It, however, did not immediately result in the establishment of any hospital.

Lock Hospitals

None of the above-mentioned hospitals treated female patients and no proposal was forthcoming for creating hospitals for female patients either. However, in his account of early hospitals in Calcutta, Dr D.G. Crawford, quoting from the *Calcutta Gazette* of 17 January 1811, mentioned that lock hospitals for the detention and treatment of prostitutes infected with venereal diseases were already well-recognized institutions in India by 1811.[12]

In the 1820s and 1830s, out of an average establishment of about 8,500 Europeans of the Bengal army, approximately 2,400 patients suffering from venereal diseases were treated in regimental hospitals each year.[13] The presence of venereal diseases among European soldiers was 'most troubling' as well as 'embarrassing' to the authorities. Of all the venereal diseases, syphilis was numerically the most significant.[14]

Soldiers and sailors remained a major source of infection for venereal disease, but, it was thought of as a disease 'that threatened the army from without, especially from contact with low caste Indian prostitutes'.[15]

A systematic effort at combating venereal diseases was started as early as in 1807, when the Bengal government sanctioned the establishment of lock hospitals at some of the principal stations of the Bengal army, including Mathura and Fatagarh.[16] By 1822, the lock hospitals at the major stations of the Bengal army collectively treated over 4,000 women a year for venereal diseases.[17] In 1828, the number of women patients rose to 4,830, who were treated at a total cost of Rs 34,383.[18] By then, there were a total of sixteen lock hospitals in Bengal.

Between 1805 and 1833 most cantonments, which housed some 26,000 European soldiers, were equipped with lock hospitals for the forcible confinement of women suspected of venereal infection. Support for lock hospitals was initially greatest amongst army officers, who sought to stem the flow of soldiers seeking medical treatment for venereal infections. By the 1830s, military officers were joined by many surgeons who had also come to view lock hospitals as a necessary and possibly unique solution to the problem of venereal diseases.

In Bengal, however, the reforming Governor General William Bentinck pointed out to the court of directors that abolition of lock hospitals would save Rs 30,000 a year.[19] The Burma War had caused tremendous strains on the Company's finances and economies were being eagerly searched out, especially within the bloated military establishments of India.[20] Subsequently, lock hospitals were abolished in Bengal in 1830. The system was discontinued elsewhere by 1835.

The establishment of lock hospitals can be analysed from the vantage point of the nexus of sexuality, gender, class, and medical discourses.[21] Hyam's interpretation of imperialism as a hydraulic, libidinal release for repressed British youth has been tempered by studies that have sought out the construction and regulation of contingent sexual relations in the social spaces of the empire.[22] Stoler has drawn upon Foucault to suggest that metropolitan sexualities were informed by imperial circuits of power and identity.[23]

In Britain, apprehensions about the moral and physical consequences of venereal diseases persuaded a number of doctors, philanthropists, and local officials that something had to be done.[24] The most common treatment for syphilis at this time was mercury. Syphilis was generally attributed to an especially virulent poison that had entered the patient's body and lodged itself in all places, and had to be driven out through the application of strong remedy. The powerful effects of mercury were attested by the patient's salivation and perspiration, which were taken as signs that the poison had left the body. Mercury was administered to the patient in three ways: orally in the shape of what were referred to as 'blue pills' (a mixture of mercury, confection of roses, and powdered licorice), as an ointment (referred to as applied by 'friction' in contemporary texts), and finally, and less commonly, as mercury vapours.[25] By the early nineteenth century, there was increasing opposition to the use of mercury in treating syphilis.[26]

Syphilis was primarily interpreted as a disease of inflammation, and, therefore, it was supposed to require an antiphlogistic regime of diet, enemas, laxatives, and occasionally bleeding, to control the irritation of the inflamed membranes.

In the absence of efficacious medical treatment, attention shifted to adoption of preventive measures. Since effective physical barriers were not present—mass-produced condoms had to await the development of vulcanized rubber and the first really affordable ones were not available until 1900[27]—efforts were directed at the carrier of the disease. Sander Gilman's work on nineteenth-century depictions of such diseases has pointed out the common practice of playing up the maleness of the sufferer, who was considered to be the incidental victim 'of the female's infection'.[28] It has been pointed out that it is no accident that the campaign to control venereal diseases through the introduction of lock hospitals in India coincided with the opening of a number of lock hospitals in Britain: Glasgow (1805), Newcastle (1813), Manchester (1819), Liverpool (1834), and Leeds (1842).[29] Lock hospitals in Britain directed their efforts not only at curing the disease, but also at dealing with the moral failings, which it was felt had led the patient to contract the disease in the first place. In Britain, however, these hospitals lacked the blatantly coercive character of their counterparts in India.

Opposition to the use of mercury for treating venereal diseases had a somewhat different dimension in India. Unlike in Western countries, anti-mercurial position in India was related to some extent to environmental perceptions of disease. As noted by Mark Harrison, colonial medical practices did not simply mimic metropolitan medicine.[30] Medical thought on the colonial periphery was heavily weighted in favour of environmental influences, and diseases were often presented as having characteristics that differed according to the part of the world in which they were experienced. As one surgeon explained, 'In tropical regions, disease is of the most acute kind and rapid in its progress.'[31] The author concluded that despite its initial ferocity, secondary or constitutional syphilis was less of a concern because hot-climate diseases do not produce the same chronic conditions found in other climates.

Many army surgeons in India were also bent on insisting that a distinction should be made between simple syphilis and complicated syphilis (or primary and secondary syphilis): only the latter required mercury. Simple syphilis, which they argued was more common in the army, was better treated without mercury for in such cases the cure, that is heavy metal poisoning, was believed to be ultimately more harmful than the disease.

Proponents of mercury, on the other hand, emphasized that since non-mercurial treatments required a much longer stay in hospital, soldiers would, therefore, be taken out of active service for longer stretches of time without there being any solid evidence to suggest that such a regime offered a better chance for recuperation. Treatments for venereal diseases tended to vary between hospitals since regimental surgeons were left free to employ whatever therapy they thought was best suited.

These diseases posed a potential threat not only to troops' physical well-being but also to the maintenance of military discipline as well, when soldiers sought sexual gratification amongst the local prostitutes residing outside the confines of the barracks. The failure to establish an effective strategy of medical intervention within the army prompted surgeons to agree with army officers that they would have to employ alternative remedies or juridical methods to counter the putative carrier—the prostitute. As pointed out by Laura Briggs, 'One of the features of modern colonial states was that their characteristic response to the problem of prostitution was bureaucratic—medical inspection, registration, and incarceration in lock hospitals.'[32] The strategy of surveillance and control applied to regulate prostitution, although not unique to India, was certainly pushed with greater zeal and *took a further twist as it was being transferred not only between the sexes but also between races.* In fact, it is reasonable to argue that medical thought and military imperatives were constantly configured and reconfigured by colonial understandings of race, class, gender, and sexuality.

The 'victims' of venereal diseases in India were commonly presented as white and male; the 'perpetrators', that is, the prostitutes, as Indian and female, and discussions on how to try and interdict transmission of the disease ranged well beyond narrow epidemiological and clinical boundaries. The production of an official position on sexuality, and its subsequent regulation, was crucial to imperial efforts to police the various hierarchies which sustained the imperial project, namely hierarchies of race, gender, and class.[33] British medical and military officers in India were white, male, and belonged to the middle if not upper class; gender and race set them apart from the Indian prostitutes, while class distinguished them from the rank and file. Also, many medical and military persons expressed the opinion that soldiers were incapable of curbing their sexual desires.

Contemporary ideas of masculinity and the constructions of Indian society that were then taking shape definitely acted as deterrents in the way of intervening directly in the soldiers' sexual activities. It was thought that any attempt to do so might undermine their heterosexuality, which the army prized so highly.

It has been argued that since masculinity became an important prism through which colonial societies could be observed and ranked, and 'the manliness of the European conqueror was set against the fickle and effeminate Indian male', nothing could be done that would jeopardize such a hierarchy and would raise any uncertainty about the European male, and 'so the soldier was left alone'.[34] No doubt, military imperatives and medical policies in India were both part of a broader moral/cultural domain, in which were inscribed the prejudices and assumptions of a masculine colonial ideology.

The Indian prostitute, like India itself, was objectified and problematized in a way that would have been inconceivable had colonial rule not produced the types of cultural and scientific discourses that legitimated the belief in an inherent difference between India and Europe, and between Indian prostitutes and European prostitutes.

Soldiers, who were thought incapable of resisting temptation at the best of times, were considered to be at even greater risk in India, where prostitution was commonly understood by the British to be a time-honoured profession with no shame attached to it. As early as 1810 one commentator was insisting that 'in every part of India the profession of a prostitute is devoid of that stigma annexed to it in Europe; persons following it are protected by law in certain privileges'.[35]

This archetype of the Indian prostitute can be partly accounted for by contemporary readings of caste and occupation which gave priority to hereditary explanations, and partly by the increasing use of sexuality and gender as important means of establishing a moral and cultural hierarchy in which Europeans ranked above Indians. As Levine has pointed out, the mere existence of a prostitute 'caste' (into which were folded commercial prostitutes as well as courtesans and temple dancers) was useful proof to the British of just how debased Indian society had become.[36] Closely coupled with this construction of the Indian prostitute was the more general idea that Indian women were inherently less able to control their sexuality, proof of just how far their environment and society had frustrated any chances of moral regeneration from within. Once again, medical proof was forthcoming to bolster these assertions. It was suggested:

> The women's diseases, we know and hear little of; but, as strictly sexual, we may infer, from their early marriages, that they will be more the diseases of debility and relaxation (diseased mammae and ovaria), than those of an opposite nature to which the female is prone in European countries.[37]

The argument that Indian prostitutes would accept genital examination with nonchalance was advanced as further proof of the degraded nature of Indian women.[38] Such representations of Indian women, which undercut their claims to a common humanity, paved the way for others who would defend the use of 'a little wholesome coercion' to combat venereal diseases in India.[39]

Some observers embedded prostitution in the social and economic structures of the subcontinent and tied the rise and fall of venereal disease to agrarian conditions. They argued that in times of famine, the number of women around stations increased, and with it venereal disease became more common. One surgeon serving in the Madras Presidency calculated the rates of infection over a seventeen-year period, and showed that the rate was highest in years of dearth. The average for the 13th Dragoons was forty cases per year, but in 1824–5 and 1833–4 (both periods of famine) the number topped one hundred. In those years, 'the poor and half starved villagers have been known to cohabitate with the men of our regiment for a handful of grain.'[40]

After the abolition of lock hospitals, the debate regarding how best to combat venereal diseases became more intense. It was calculated that of the European troops stationed in Madras between 1829 and 1838, one-third of the hospital admissions were for syphilis.[41] John Hall, the Inspector General of Hospitals in Bombay, computed that in a 12-month period (April 1851 to April 1852), there were 414 cases of syphilis (primary and secondary), 54 cases of penile ulcers, 202 cases of bubos, and 301 gonorrhoeal cases.[42]

The difficulty of mobilizing support for the reopening of lock hospitals was considerably eased in the 1830s by the appearance, in that decade, of a growing number of professional publications through which army officers and medical surgeons could air their opinions.[43] The physical health, moral condition, and efficiency of soldiers provided a site upon which these professional agendas could overlap, and venereal diseases were a frequent subject of articles and letters to the editors in both the military press and in medical periodicals.

In the wake of the indigenous rebellion of 1857, direct rule and the scaling back of the numbers of local Indian militia had led to the arrival in India of unprecedented masses of British troops. After 1860 or so, imperial policy dictated the permanent maintenance of a force of some 60,000 regular British soldiers, roughly double the number stationed in India before 1857.[44] The presence of so substantial a contingent of men, mostly young and single as well as of predominantly working-class origin, saw the growth of a distinctive barracks culture in which recreational sex, primarily with local women, became increasingly commonplace.[45] Though sexual contacts between indigenous women and foreign colonizing men were by no means new, the expanded presence of British soldiers certainly increased such connection.

It is worth mentioning that before 1857, managing prostitution was not seen as the only solution to containing venereal disease in the European army. Concubinage with Indian women among white soldiers was encouraged by the colonial medical bureaucracy as an effective means of curbing venereal disease.[46] It was considered to be a possible option not only for curbing venereal diseases, but also for increasing the efficiency of the army. The Indian Medical Board commented in 1810: 'Inducements might be held out to the men to attach themselves individually to individual Native women, [since] it [is] well known, how much more efficient those Corps are, which have native women attached to them.'[47]

After the rebellion of 1857, concubinage became suspect as disloyal. Indian prostitutes were increasingly described as belonging to a separate caste.[10] In the changed atmosphere of the post-1857 era—which saw the influx of a large number of troops to the Indian subcontinent—improvement of army health became an even more major area of concern.

The ratio of British to Indian troops had been increased so as to bolster security, but this investment could only be fruitful if the European soldiers were kept free of venereal diseases. The Royal Commission into the Sanitary State of the Army in India (1863), however, found out that this was not the case, as a result of which the lock hospital system was regularized and extended through the Cantonment Act (XXII of 1864).

Combining the United Kingdom's established emphasis on visibility with an 'orientalist sociology', the Indian Cantonment Act divided prostitutes into those who were and were not frequented by Europeans, with only the former coming under regulation.[49] Ballhatchet has shown that these women were registered within the cantonment, examined every month, and detained in a lock hospital if infected.[50]

Cantonment Acts

There was also a more complex geography that the Cantonment Act created. It demanded a sophisticated system of surveillance such that the spaces and subjects under its purview were divided and statistically surveyed.[51] It has also been suggested that the Cantonment Acts represent the disciplining of public space through surveillance, in conformity with Foucault's four arts of distributions (enclosure, partition, function, and rank).[52] These spaces of surveillance were created, first, through enclosing public prostitutes away from 'normal' Indian women. While Indian women were regularly suspected of promiscuity or immorality in official reports, prostitutes were set apart as being both socially lascivious and politically dangerous in terms of their effect on British military power. This is reflected in the first categorization of the Cantonment Act that questioned whether a prostitute was frequented or not by Europeans, with non-registered prostitutes being expelled from the cantonment.

Within this enclosed area there would be no public soliciting on the threat of arrest, and any woman suspected of being a non-registered prostitute could be reported. The Act also gave the Cantonment Committee the authority to extend their powers beyond the enclosure if other prostitutes were readily available to the soldiers. Within the enclosure, space was then partitioned into registered homes, which could be inspected at will and maintained to a degree of cleanliness dictated by the Cantonment Committee.[53]

Information gathered from these enclosed and partitioned women was collected in centres of calculation, at both the cantonment magistrate's office and the office of the lock hospital. The surveyed bodies were given a function, through reading the rules to the prostitutes when they registered, and giving them a copy of the regulations in their language such that their function as healthy, docile bodies was made clear. Finally, the women were ranked through fortnightly examinations, the results of which were kept in a register and on the woman's ticket, with infected women being forcibly incarcerated in the lock hospital until cured.

In Bengal, the rate of admissions of soldiers suffering from venereal diseases rose from 177 per 1,000 men in 1855 to 359 in 1859.[54] In official circles, there was anxiety about the spread of the disease among not only soldiers, but also sailors in Calcutta. According to medical practitioners like Dr Ferris (of Messrs Scott, Thomson and Company) '*not less than 20 per cent* of seamen that visit this port are inoculated with some form of syphilitic disease'.[55] J.A. Crawford, collector of customs, for example, pointed out:

> There is no question that sailors require as much, if not almost more, care in this respect than soldiers. The latter are almost always within reach of treatment; I may say always, for they have the regimental Surgeons to whom to apply at once.

He further noted that unlike soldiers, sailors could not get this attention. 'A case within my own knowledge occurred in which the sufferer left Calcutta via the Cape of Good Hope for England. The disease did not show itself till St. Helena was reached, and the victim died some days before the coast of England was sighted.'[56]

Many in India were in favour of introduction of legislation like the English C.D. Act for curbing venereal diseases.[57] Crawford, for instance, stated: 'The best means of prevention would be the enforcement of the C.D. Act. No legislation will be of any effect, unless the root of the evil is reached; and this cannot be done unless there is a registration of the prostitutes in each port, and then compulsory subjection of them to medical examination.'[58]

Medical opinion sometimes also showed concern about the spread of syphilitic diseases amongst all classes of the population, Christian and native.[59] According to one estimate, more than 30,000 women in Calcutta were entirely dependent on prostitution for their maintenance and support, and many of them no doubt catered to the needs of the European population of the town. Reportedly, syphilitic diseases existed among the public prostitutes of the town in the following ratio: Hindu women of high caste: 15 per cent; Hindu women of inferior caste: 30 per cent; Muslim and low-caste Hindu women: 50 per cent; and low Christians and other nondescript prostitutes: 5 per cent. The last two classes of women who resided in Jaun Bazaar, Bow Bazaar, and Champatolla were frequented mostly by soldiers and sailors.[60]

Eventually, in 1868, the colonial authorities in India enacted the C.D. Act of 1868 (Act XIV, or Chaudda Ain). Unlike the earlier attempts at controlling prostitution before the 1860s, which affected only women consorting with soldiers, the new legislation extended control beyond the military horizon by introducing regulation in the Presidencies. The extension of the Act in 1864 can be interpreted to mean that after the mid-nineteenth century, this link was becoming powerful. According to Ashis Nandy, before 1830, when middle-class mores were less powerful, this sexual–political link was less apparent.[61] Violations of the provisions of the Act of 1868 would lead to the arrest of the offenders. The Act could be introduced in any locality specified by a local government, with the sanction of the governor general.[62] Initially, it was proposed that four lock hospitals be established in Calcutta. Till the 1870s, apparently two lock hospitals—one at Alipore, and the other at Sealdah—were functioning.[63]

The operation of the Indian C.D. Act was more stringent than that of the British Act. Unlike the British C.D. Acts, which required a police officer to swear before a magistrate that a woman was a common prostitute in order for her to be subjected to medical check-up for signs of venereal disease, under the C.D. Act in India, prostitutes had to register with authorities, then volunteer for routine medical examinations. In Calcutta, the Act's administration was entrusted to the ordinary local police. Moreover, every police officer was authorized to arrest, even without warrant, any common prostitute who had failed to appear for registration or to attend the examination.

The medical examination of registered prostitutes was conducted daily, Sundays excepted. A system of private home examination for women who would apply for it, and agree to pay Rs 4 per month for the privilege, was also officially sanctioned. The house-visiting system, however, was only acceptable to the higher classes of prostitutes who were prepared to pay the fee. Around 1869–70, there were 227 women under home examination, of whom only 0.3 per cent were suffering from diseases. Most of these women were of a class almost above the rank of common prostitutes.

The annual report of the superintendent of lock hospitals on the working of the C.D. Act in 1872 pointed out that at the close of the year, the total number of women on the registers was 6,871, as against 7,087 on 31 December 1871, showing a decrease of 216 names. Among those named, Hindus were the majority, numbering around 5,804, followed by Muslims (930), East Indians (85), Russians and Wallachians (20), Poles (11), Austrians (8), Hungarians (3), Italians (3), French (2), English (2), Irish (2), and Spaniards (1). The decrease was caused because thirty-one names were removed from the registers after exemption from the operation of the Act, while 56 died and 436 women were lost sight of.

The elaborate operations under the Act can be understood from the facts furnished by the official reports regarding the arrest of defaulters, statistical information regarding imprisonment, and so on. In 1873, 103 women were arrested for non-registration; 97 were registered after arrest; 5 were fined; 1 was imprisoned; 2,862 were arrested as defaulters from examination; 2,661 were warned by the commissioner; 47 were warned by a magistrate; 53 were fined by a magistrate; and 101 were imprisoned by a magistrate.[64] It is known from the lock hospital superintendent's annual report on the working of the C.D. Act in 1873 we know that in that year the number of women on the register liable to attend examination was 6,455, against 6,871 in 1872. Of them, there were 5,435 Hindus, 891 Muslims, 88 East Indians, 21 Russians and Wallachians, 2 Austrians, 7 Poles, 3 Hungarians, 2 Italians, 2 French, 1 Spaniard, and 3 English.

The contested nature of the medical opinion regarding the effectiveness of the Act is shown by the fact that while noting the extent of the success of the Act, it was also mentioned that total eradication of venereal diseases could not be achieved only through this enactment. Around 1873, satisfaction was expressed by S.M. Shircore, superintendent of lock hospitals in Calcutta, about the working of the Act, which resulted in 'great benefit to the health of both the male population of Calcutta and its suburbs and the registered women themselves'.[65] At the same time, it was also pointed out that it would be very difficult to completely eradicate venereal disease even with the very best supervision and control over women, because the increase of venereal complaints was affected by causes that lay beyond the scope of the Act. On 25 March 1873, S.M. Shircore wrote to the commissioner of police:

> I seek permission to point out a common error in connection with the working of the C.D. Act which seems to prevail pretty generally. There is an idea that among other good effects which must necessarily follow the introduction of the Act ought to be a complete eradication of all kinds of venereal diseases in Calcutta. But those who anticipate such results forget that while the women are subjected to supervision and periodical examinations in order to protect the male population from contamination no protection whatever is afforded them against their being infected by the opposite sex. There are hundreds of men who arrive in Calcutta daily from various parts of the world, and there is no doubt that a large proportion of them import and spread disease, the worst among them being the sailors. As long as such source of infection continues to exist, it would be unreasonable to expect a complete disappearance of these diseases.[66]

Around 1881, the high court and the police magistrate made two important decisions which seemed to affect the working of the C.D. Act. In the case of one Nistarini Raur, it was decided that any woman who petitioned to have her name removed from the register was entitled to have it removed. Moreover, the police were fined for arresting two women, Kusom and Attur, without a warrant, the legality of such arrest being denied by the magistrate. After this decision, arrests without warrants were discontinued.[67] Subsequently, by the government notification of 1 October 1881, published in the *Calcutta Gazette* on 5 October 1881, the operation of the Act was limited from 1 November of that year to a smaller area in the southern part of Calcutta and its suburbs. The examination wards at Chitpore and Bowbazar were abolished. It was decided to restrict the limits of the Act to that part of the town inhabited by women who received soldiers, and to confine its operation to the protection of the military alone.[68]

According to Sir Ashley Eden, the then governor general of India, police atrocities, which made the Act unpopular among a large section of the public and the press, and legal complications arising out of the ruling of the Calcutta High Court, which declared the act's rules of procedure to be illegal, necessitated this measure.

Of the 6,565 women on the register on 31 October 1881, the names of 4,604 women who were residing beyond the modified limits were struck off from the roll, leaving a balance of 1,961 women within these limits. Of this number, about 1,010 women, who were known to be willing to receive visits from soldiers, were required to undergo medical examination. For the remainder, it was optional, and practically all of them gave up attendance.

The only effectual power that seemed to be retained under the Act was that of arresting those women whose names were on the register and who failed to attend examination. The percentage of arrests of defaulters during 1881 was around 64, against 83 in 1880, and cases of disease discovered among them fell from about 9 per cent in 1880 to around 5 per cent in 1881.[69] Over the years, those who suffered from syphilis included women of many professions, who perhaps combined prostitution with other things. In March 1883, Surgeon General Nicholson, officiating super of lock hospitals, presented to the commissioner of police, Calcutta, the following list of patients who were suffering from syphilis (see Table 1.1).

By the early 1880s, it was becoming quite evident that the experiment with lock hospitals had not been very effective in checking the spread of venereal diseases among British troops. It was observed in 1884 that in the Bengal Presidency as a whole, the annual average ratio of admissions from venereal disease per 1,000 was just what it had been in 1863,

Table 1.1 Patients with Syphilis (1883)

Name	Alleged occupation
Atar	Prostitute
Golap	Day labourer
Prosunno	Beggar
Koolashi	Maid servant
Prosunno	Coolie
Tara	Nil
Ananta	Beggar
Dukhini	Day labourer
Ruman	Maid servant
Fulmoney	Nil

Source: Proceedings of the Government of Bengal General Department, 1883.

twenty-one years earlier, when there were no lock hospitals. Excepting 1878, when the ratio reached 288 per 1,000, the rate for 1883 was higher than it had been in any year since 1862, when it equalled 318 per 1,000.[70]

The annual average ratio of admissions of women suffering from venereal diseases per 1,000 women was 281 in 1863 (before the enactment of C.D. Act), and more or less remained the same during the next twenty years. Yet, around the same period, the incidence of venereal diseases among the troops in India rose from 196.8 per 1,000 in 1871 to 342.7 per 1,000 in 1885. In the heart of Calcutta itself, in Fort William (where the soldiers were supposed to be the most protected, and the prostitutes serving them were regularly examined), the percentage of cases of venereal diseases was found to have risen to 14.5 in 1882—higher than it had been in any year since the introduction of the C.D. Act. This, no doubt, strengthened the case of those who condemned the C.D. Act.

The Indian press condemned the Act as 'a useless piece of legislation' and also criticized its oppressive nature.[71] The pressure to abolish it mounted after the repeal of the British C.D. Act in 1886.[72] The Indian C.D. Act was ultimately abolished in 1888.

The working of the lock hospitals and of the C.D. Act showed how the question of medically managing the relationship between soldiers, sailors, and Indian prostitutes produced a particular configuration of class and race, and was also controlled by it. It may be further suggested, as pointed out by Ashis Nandy, that 'the homology between sexual and political dominance which Western colonialism invariably used...was not an accidental by-product of colonial history' but an integral clue to the workings of colonialism.[73]

The contestations over registration and medical examination showed that Indian prostitutes were regarded as belonging to a separate class. Whereas under the British C.D. Act, English women were treated as involved in a criminal act, Indian women were thought to be belonging to a separate class, 'of being (ontologically and essentially) prostitutes'. Moreover, prostitutes for 'English use' were not supposed to engage in sex with Indian men. In this sense also, they were constituted as belonging to a particular kind of class, which was monitored not only for disease, but for maintaining some peculiar kind of racial purity.[74]

Right from the start, treatment at the lock hospitals was marked by racial discrimination. Officials seemed to be sympathetic to the non-Indian prostitutes who expressed annoyance for being detained among natives in the examining wards. According to the commissioner of police, Calcutta, this factor 'is certainly regarded by them as the most unpleasant part of registration under the Act'.[75] It was suggested that arrangements be made for setting apart one day for the examination of European or Eurasian women only. Subsequently, in November 1873, native patients were removed to the Alipore Lock Hospital and the accommodation at Sealdah was reserved for European and Eurasian women only.

Apart from reinforcing the societal class and racist norms by segregating patients through the practice of curative medicine, another historical feature related to the working of the C.D. Act was the lack of efficaciousness of medical treatment delivered to suspected patients. As pointed out by Geraldine Forbes: 'Infected women were sent to lock hospitals and treated, often with mercury, until the symptoms disappeared.' She also writes: 'The records indicate women resisted these examinations as well as the entire system of registration, while officials complained that *dhais* hired to carry out the distasteful inspections were in collusion with the prostitutes.'[76] The common prostitutes were subjected to different kinds of crude and obnoxious medical examinations and were kept under filthy conditions. Indian women found these hospitals revolting to their habits and customs. The indigenous curative means, which were known for years or ages, were held in high estimation; however, this might not be the case if they were found to be less efficacious than those employed by the Europeans.[77]

According to official opinion, every prostitute would try their utmost to evade registration. Throughout the 1870s and till its repeal in 1888, at least twelve women on an average were arrested daily for violation of the rules.[78] The number of arrests of defaulters increased from 1,775 in 1871 to 2,303 in 1872.[79] Admissions into the hospitals, however, increased from 2,037 to 2,941 in 1872. The C.D. Act (and the lock hospitals), no doubt, was meant to organize 'disorderly' women, 'often limiting their mobility to segregated districts, enrolling them as imperial citizens through the essentially bureaucratic process of registration, and sometimes restricting their clients by race'.[80] It has also been argued that the impact of the contagious diseases legislation in India introduced 'a new form of bodily regulation', in which the moral division between respectable and unrespectable women in India began to be detached from a sacred social hierarchy and came to be expressed through Western medical metaphors of health and disease. Moreover, lock hospitals were regarded as institutions for treating the so-called unclean bodies of prostitutes.[81]

Hospital Care and Female Patients

While lock hospitals served only prostitutes, other women were meant to be given medical attention through lying-in hospitals. Official records tell us that the earliest lying-in hospital in Calcutta was established in 1814 'under the auspices of the Right Honourable the Countess of Loudon and Moira'.[82] It seems that it took more than two decades for another such hospital to be established in Calcutta. In fact, from the 1840s, a number of maternity hospitals were established not only in Calcutta but also in some other Indian towns. It has been rightly pointed out that these hospitals—which were aimed at a population that had no direct bearing on colonial rule—had symbolic importance.[83] Undoubtedly, 'as beacons of humanity and enlightenment, it was hoped that they would contrast sharply with the "darkness" of Indian society and its treatment of women'.[84] It can further be suggested that they also led to more and more medicalization of female bodies, albeit slowly, and along with it created a demand for medical care that was patterned on the Western, and supposedly advanced, form of medicine, where women were to be involved both as patients, and (later) as care givers.

In 1840, a large female (lying-in) hospital containing 100 beds was constructed on the grounds of the CMC by public subscription.[85] It provided training to male medical professionals in the use of modern techniques, including forceps and ether, to make deliveries easier. The prospectus mentioned that a high rate of mortality prevailed among 'lower orders of female population during parturition', which 'chiefly affects the females of the Christian and Jewish religions.'[86] The hospital also afforded instructions in midwifery.[87] The European matron who taught the students under the general direction of the professor of midwifery was expected to follow the system pursued at the lying-in hospitals of Paris, London, and Dublin.[88]

Women patients were generously offered gifts 'in the shape of clothes for themselves and their children when they left'. They also received 'an allowance for tobacco and such like indulgences, while in the hospital.'[89] In 1852, a large hospital, which was designed to accommodate 350 patients, was opened.[90] One hundred and sixteen beds were reserved for women and children. Fifty of these beds were placed under the charge of the professor of midwifery and were devoted to pregnancy and diseases associated with it.[91]

Attendance at the outpatient department for diseases of women and children increased in the 1860s. Dr S.B. Patridge, officiating principal of Medical College, wrote to Dr Hugh Macpherson, secretary to the principal inspector general, medical department: 'In the out-patient Department (also) the attendance at the Dispensary, for the diseases of women and children, has been greater than usual; the excess over the attendance in 1860 amounting to no less than 1,917.'[92] He also believed that the popularity of the 'Sub-Division of the Hospital' was due to 'the appointment of a steady married man as Resident House Surgeon.'[93]

The official report of 1877 recorded the number of female patients (and also sometimes children) treated in different medical institutions in the city of Calcutta as well as the suburbs. Institutions included were: Medical College Hospital, General Hospital, Mayo Hospital and Dispensaries, Campbell Hospital, Municipal Police Hospital (these were Calcutta hospitals), North Suburban Hospital, Sumbhoonath

Pundit Dispensary, Alipore Dispensary, Arratoon Apcar Dispensary, and Howrah General Hospital (known as Suburban Hospital). The number of female patients treated in different hospitals in Calcutta and the suburbs rose from 49,076 in 1876 to 49,798 in 1877.[94] Despite this rise, when compared with the admission of men, admission of women in hospitals was a rare phenomenon. The proportion of male to female adults admitted to hospitals for treatment was reported to be about four to one in 1880. A total of 1,63,925 adult males and 15,584 adult females were treated in different medical institutions in Calcutta. Of them, 40,563 adult males and 4,298 females were in-patients. The death rate among adults was 138.6 and among children 133.[95]

By 1842, six dispensaries had been established in Bengal.[96] Around 1867 there were sixty-one dispensaries. The number rose to over 500 in 1900. According to modern researchers, although the number of women attending dispensaries rose by the turn of the century, it was 'simply a function of the growing number of such institutions in the province'.[97] The attendance of female patients in Calcutta medical institutions, no doubt, remained far below the expectations of officials and physicians. On the other hand, admission to hospitals itself did not guarantee proper treatment and cure for the patients. In fact, for a long time, mortality in hospitals continued to be quite high. People often died from primary and secondary haemorrhage, tetanus, erysepelas, gangrene, septicaemia, and exhaustion.[98] Reasons for hospitalization, which apparently included 'sloughing, gangrene, erysipelas, pleuresy, pericarditis, empyema, peritonitis and all cases of septicaemia', were responsible for 31.06 per cent of mortality in the Medical College Hospitals between 1864 and 1869.[99] The advent of Listerism in Great Britain in the 1870s aroused tremendous interest among practitioners in Calcutta.[100] The effectiveness of the application of Lister's method of anti-sepsis in controlling hospitalization, however, remained a debatable issue. The report of the Calcutta Medical College Hospital for the year 1880 contained two communications of Dr Kenneth McLeod, the first surgeon, and of Dr D.O'C. Raye, second surgeon, who expressed divergent opinions about the value of Listerism. Surgeon General Dr A.J. Payne came to the conclusion that 'Listerism has not yet established its claim to infallibility or the precise degree of its superiority over other treatments'.[101] Dr Kenneth McLeod himself went to Edinburgh in

1876, saw Lister's work, and after returning to India in 1879, attempted to introduce it in an improved form. He also published an annual précis of operations in the *Indian Medical Gazette* (*IMG*) to record the diminishing incidence of sepsis. Through his constant efforts and advocacy of 'strict' Listerism, the use of antiseptic seemed to have become an established fact by 1885.[102]

Nursing for patients, another important ingredient of health care service provided in institutions, developed slowly over the years. The successful employment of female nurses by the government in the Military Hospital at Allahabad during the Rebellion of 1857 gave an impetus to the development of nursing in Calcutta hospitals. Supported by Lady Canning, the wife of the first viceroy of India, and also encouraged by Dr Forsyth, the then inspector general of hospitals, and Dr Eatwell, principal of the CMC, the Calcutta Hospital Nurses' Institution adopted different measures aimed at fostering medical care by trained female nurses in the Calcutta hospitals.[103]

Changing Nature of Health Care: From Bedside Medicine to Hospital Medicine

The East India Company's rule in India was contemporaneous with momentous changes and advancement in the theory and practice of medicine in the West. Scholars who have studied the evolution of hospital medicine amongst the Western nations have drawn our attention to the fact that the advent of clinical medicine, along with the changes which accompanied it, eventually led to the growth of a new paradigm of knowledge and brought about important transformations in the nature of medical care. The growth of medical institutions, including clinics and teaching hospitals in British India as well, meant that health care practices were undergoing important changes, with significant outcome for both male and female patients.

E. Ackerknecht, in his study of Parisian hospitals, identified the hospital, together with the techniques which were associated with it—physical examination, autopsy, and statistics—as the basis for a new form of medicine which swept across Europe in the late eighteenth and early nineteenth centuries.[104] Thus, there started a far-reaching transformation from pre-hospital bedside medicine to hospital medicine around the late eighteenth century. Apparently, the new public hospitals accepted patients from lowly backgrounds and appointed relatively high-status physicians to treat them. According to Waddington, who accepted Ackerknecht's analysis of the importance of the hospital in the development of modern medicine, this shift meant a movement of medicine from upper-class client control to medical dominance.

Three years later, N. Jewson presented a different analysis of the link between medical knowledge and the extant form of social relationships.[105] Medicine, which dominated western Europe from the Middle ages until the late eighteenth century, was available to minority groups such as rich people, who would chose those doctors whom they believed could help them most. During the phase of bedside medicine, the patients themselves could define the nature of illness. But the advent of hospital medicine meant that the doctor's role became dominant, which, in its turn, ensured 'the emergence of a medicine based on pathological lesions which were inaccessible to the patient without medical interpretation'.[106] According to some researchers, 'The Marxist notion of alienation is clearly recognizable in Jewson's thesis that the move to Hospital Medicine marked "the disappearance of the sick man from hospital cosmologies"'.[107]

Michel Foucault in his works, particularly in *The Birth of the Clinic* and *Discipline and Punish: The Birth of the Prison*,[108] provided another framework for understanding the growth and nature of clinical practice. Like many authors, Foucault also believed that the eighteenth century saw, among other things, 'the emergence of a clinical medicine strongly centred on individual examination, diagnosis and therapy'.[109] As Alan Sheridan points out in his translator's note to *The Birth of the Clinic*, by 'clinic' Foucault meant both the clinical method and the teaching hospital.[110] Foucault also situated the attempted reforms of hospitals in late eighteenth century within a complex framework of growth of new policies. For Foucault, changes in the field of medicine were part of a wider cognitive revolution. Just like diseases, bodies that contained the disease were also sought to be produced by a range of techniques deployed through different disciplinary institutions like hospitals, prisons workshops, and so on. Disciplinary power became the new, more dominant and pervasive power mechanism than sovereign power, which now operated through developing the new techniques of body. Foucault analysed Bentham's concept of the panopticon as the main exemplar of the new power mechanism or the new principle of surveillance. In the prison as well as the hospital, bodies were observed and analysed. The clinic became a centre where large numbers of non-resistant populations passed under the gaze of a relatively few clinicians and their students, who were socialized into the way of seeing and the social order that attended their increasing status.

Following Russell Maulitz, scholars like Mark Harrison point out that compared to France, which witnessed great advancement in pathological anatomy, in Britain it 'appears to have been of interest only to a relatively small minority of medical practitioners, most of whom were concentrated in Edinburgh and London'.[111] Moreover, it has been convincingly argued by Harrison that the classic features of 'clinical' or 'hospital' medicine were present in India prior to 1800. The steady supply of cadavers, absence of constraints upon dissection, and unification of surgical and medical practices led to the refinement of an organ-based pathology into a pathology of tissues, and also encouraged British surgeons who worked in the environment of colonial hospitals in India to attempt to correlate post-mortem findings with bedside observations. Eventually, the observations made in these hospitals and in post-mortem examinations provided the foundation of medical practice in India.[112] Surgeons like James Johnson and William Twining even theorized about differences between European and Indian bodies based on post-mortem observations. It is interesting to note that Twining, and before him John Clark, remarked about the more adverse physical impact of Indian climate on European women compared to Indian women. Twining observed that hysteria was rare among Indian women because of 'the modified scale of sympathies' between the body and the climate, which saved Indians from many of the complaints that afflicted Europeans.[113]

With the establishment of hospitals in India by the British, Indian patients, who were so far treated within their domestic settings, began to experience a new era of being interned within the hospital for medical help and treatment. After the foundation of the Medical College in Calcutta in 1835, anatomical dissection was introduced in medical curricula. The act of cadaveric dissection brought about changes in the perception of the body, health, and illness, and an altogether different paradigm of knowledge emerged in the Indian context. Indigenous knowledge of the body and health was made marginal. Arguably, the lack of precise anatomical knowledge in Āyurvedic texts was the fundamental reason for its giving way to Western medical superiority. Anatomy came to be regarded as the scientific cornerstone for the study of medicine. Since the performance of the first dissection by Madhusudan Gupta and four other Indians in 1836, practical anatomy made rapid progress. Between 1837 and 1847, the Medical College was supplied with 3,500 Indian bodies for dissection.[114] It gradually developed a first-class pathological museum and also recruited local artists to produce plates as well as demonstrators of anatomy. All of these were provided within two or three years after the first dissection. This, along with almost an unlimited supply of cadavers, placed the CMC 'in the top rank of teaching anatomy in the world'.[115]

Undoubtedly, the transition from bedside medicine to hospital medicine meant that a space was created—through institutionalization of Western therapies—for the legitimization of medical intervention over individual bodies. Although there were no hospitals exclusively for female patients, records of a mesmeric hospital (as noted earlier) serving peasant women, lock hospitals for treatment of female prostitutes, and lying-in hospitals for teaching purposes not only lend credibility to the argument that hospitals were established to give relief to the labouring sections, but also show that female bodies were subsequently brought under the medical gaze, albeit in a limited way. Expansion of curative medicine, accompanied by growth of surgery, midwifery, and other medical practices led to more and more medicalization of (not only male but also) female bodies. Physiological discussions regarding the woman's body, which were taking place by the mid-nineteenth century, were aided by pathological specimens located in the museum of the CMC. In his book *Pathologica Indica* published in 1848, Allan Webb, the curator of the museum of the CMC, located the various morbid specimens in their cultural context. He noted the morbid state of the sexual and reproductive organs of native women and the cultural pathologies that these lesions represented.

From the 1880s, the lying-in hospitals and missionary institutions catering to women were supplemented by hospitals staffed by female doctors from the semi-official Dufferin Fund (or the National Association for Supplying Female Medical Aid to the Women of India). As pointed out by M. Harrison, the impetus behind the scheme was not simply the humanitarian desire to extend medical relief to Indian women (primarily of the higher castes), but to inculcate Western values, especially principles of hygiene. It was thought that women held the key to improving domestic sanitation and hygienic education of the population in general.

***

As noted earlier, the quantitative impact of hospital medicine on female patients was not very noteworthy. The majority of the female (as well as male) population continued to be served by women as well as male practitioners of traditional Indian therapies. During the advent of British rule in India, health needs of women were met by midwives who had acquired commendable professional skills, as well as elderly female members of the household possessing knowledge and expertise in traditional healing methods. As discussed elsewhere, there existed a vigorous female domain of healing in early nineteenth-century Calcutta.[116]

One very famous female practitioner of traditional medicine in early nineteenth-century Calcutta was popularly known as 'Jodu's mother'.[117] She was the wife of Kasinath Datta, fourth son of Bhabanicharan Datta, who was employed as diwan in the East India Company's Public Works Department. Reportedly, Kasinath learnt about the treatment of many difficult diseases from a sage whom he met in Benaras and started practising as a medicine man in Calcutta. He taught his wife about these methods of treatment and remedies; she took up her husband's profession after his death and became an expert and popular healer. The CMC was established not long before her death and there were only a handful of Western practitioners at that time, who were apparently surprised to find her commendable skill in doctoring. Her expertise became a subject of pride for educated Calcuttans. Poet Iswarchandra Gupta even wrote a poem mentioning how she succeeded in such difficult cases where even reputed doctors and kabirajs failed to heal the patients. Another famous 'name' among women healers was 'Raju's mother', who belonged to the barber caste. She was an expert in surgery and earned a comfortable livelihood from practising surgery. Male practitioners of traditional indigenous medicine were also consulted for treating female patients.

As pointed out by Rosemary Fitzgerald,[118] colonial assumptions that Indian men, as a homogenized totality, were invariably callous and uncaring towards the health and well-being of women, were contradicted in the experiences of some missionaries. Many of the Christian missionaries, who were among the earliest outsiders to criticize the deplorable health condition of Indian women, acknowledged that Indian women depended on traditional caregivers who were accessible and acceptable to their clientele and had far stronger popular appeal than alien substitutes.

Colonial medical discourse and practice in nineteenth-century British India, no doubt, ultimately privileged Western medicine based on the knowledge of human anatomy gathered from dissection over indigenous medical systems. As the nineteenth century progressed and Western medicine received patronage from the rulers, education in scientific medicine and its dissemination was regarded as a cornerstone of the civilizing mission and underscored the colonizers' cultural authority. It meant that the domain of traditional medicine (and of traditional caregivers) was gradually discredited and marginalized in official medical policies. Along with the growth and development of hospital medicine in the course of the nineteenth century, traditional healing practices were castigated as unscientific and inadequate in the colonial rhetoric.

Saving the lives of mothers and children was not only a humanitarian goal, it was also a political one. This claim aimed at winning support from an enlightened public as well as from bureaucrats who, in the eighteenth century, were convinced that a large and healthy population was the basis for the economic, fiscal, and military strength of states. This kind of reasoning helped to make available public money for the founding of lying-in hospitals in many German states—and in other countries—during the second half of the eighteenth century. According to this view, there was a critical need for maternity hospitals in order to provide practical clinical training alongside theoretical instruction to medical students. It can be added that in India, by expanding the knowledge horizon (of physicians), it consequently gave a boost to the growth of an urge for modernizing female health care by applying biomedicine.

While traditional medical care served a more important role for a larger portion of the male as well as female populations, a clamour for the expansion of modernization of female health care—by applying biomedicine—became an inextricable part of the history of the institutionalization of curative medicine in the colonial period.

One striking feature of hospital admissions throughout India was that the proportion of women to men patients changed little over the years. Statistics sometimes even showed a decline in the number of female patients being admitted to hospitals. Mark Harrison, for example, points out that despite an overall increase in the number of patients between 1877 and 1891, 23.8 per cent of J.J. Hospital's patients in 1877 were women, and in 1891 the percentage was 21.4.[119]

The attendance of female patients in Calcutta medical institutions remained far below expectations. Although the number of women patients attending hospitals and dispensaries was rising gradually, still very few actually attended medical institutions. Low attendance of women patients (that too, only from poorer classes for a long period) gave a boost to the prevailing notion that in the conservative Indian society, women, particularly those belonging to higher social ranks, would avoid treatment by male physicians. Thus, there was a general opinion among cross sections of the population that women in India were averse to treatment by male physicians and, therefore, creation of trained female physicians was urgently needed to attend to their health needs. This logically led to a demand for the extension of medical education among women. Despite the fact that the new medical knowledge and practice were not affordable to the majority of the population, there was no demand for enhancing the opportunities of traditional caregivers. In fact, their role was gradually marginalized as they were discredited in the British civilizational discourses on science and progress. Many Indian reformers as well as British observers and administrators argued that Indian women would only accept treatment from female doctors and that they should not be deprived of the fruits of Western scientific progress. This eventually led to an expansion of demand for opening up of medical education for women, which resulted in the emergence of a group of educated women medics.

Notes and References

1. W. Ridsdale, *Record of Cases Treated in the Mesmeric Hospital—From June to December, 1847* (Calcutta: Military Orphan Press, 1848), p. 27.

2. See Waltraud Ernst, 'Under the Influence in British India: Esdaile & the Critics of His "Mesmeric Hospital" in Calcutta', *Psychological Medicine* 25 (1995): 1113–23.

3. *Centenary Volume of Calcutta Medical College* (Calcutta: 1935), p. 134.

4. *Centenary Volume of Calcutta Medical College*, p. 135.

5. The use of ether as a surgical antiseptic was developed in the 1840s in America and Europe. Later, it was challenged by the safer chloroform. See Roy Porter, 'Hospitals and Surgery', in *The Cambridge History of Medicine*, edited by Roy Porter (New York: Cambridge University Press, 2006), pp. 176–210.

6. *Centenary Volume of Calcutta Medical College*, p. 135.

7. Quoted in C.R. Wilson, 'The First Two Hospitals in Calcutta', *Indian Medical Gazette* 39, no. 1 (January 1903): 1, from Alexander Hamilton, *A New Account of the East Indies*, vol. 2 (London: 1744), p. 9. Cited in Anil Kumar, *Medicine and the Raj: British Medical Policy in India, 1835–1911* (New Delhi: SAGE Publications, 1998), p. 95.

8. Waltraud Ernst, 'The Establishment of "Native Lunatic Asylums" in Early Nineteenth-Century British India', in *Studies in Indian Medical History*, edited by G.J. Meulenbeld and D. Wujastyk (New Delhi: Motilal Banarsidass, 2001, revised edition), pp. 169–204.

9. 'Printed Proceedings of the Governors of Native Hospital dated 20th May 1835, with notes and proceedings of the General Committee from 18th June 1835 to 12th November 1840', bound manuscript volume, vol. 1, West Bengal State Archives [hereafter Fever Hospital Committee], pp. 23–4.

10. Charles Lushington, *The History, Design and Present State of the Religious, Benevolent and Charitable Institutions; Founded by the British in Calcutta and Its Vicinity* (Calcutta: Hindostanee Press, 1824).

11. Fever Hospital Committee, vol. 1, p. 24. Cited in Partha Datta, 'Ranald Martin's Medical Topography (1837): The Emergence of Public Health in Calcutta', in *The Social History of Health and Medicine in Colonial India*, edited by Mark Harrison and Biswamoy Pati (London and New York: Routledge, 2009), p. 18.

12. For some of the noteworthy studies that deal with venereal diseases, prostitution, lock hospitals, and other related subjects in the context of India, see note 35 of the Introduction.

13. In the nineteenth century, 'venereal diseases' was applied as a generic term for those diseases which were sexually transmitted. These would include what today would be identified as syphilis, gonorrhea, and a range of penile cancers. The presence of venereal diseases among European soldiers was 'most troubling' as well as 'embarrassing' to the authorities. Of all the venereal diseases, syphilis was numerically the most significant.

14. Syphilis or *firungi rog* was introduced by the Portuguese in India. Its remedy, China root, was mentioned in Bhava Misra's *Bhava Prakasa*, which is assigned to the sixteenth century. See Irfan Habib, 'Inside and Outside the Systems: Change and Innovation in Medical and Surgical Practice in Mughal India', in D. Kumar, *Disease and Medicine in India*, p. 73.

15. David Arnold, *Colonizing the Body: State Medicine and Epidemic Disease in Nineteenth-Century India* (Berkeley, California: University of California Press, 1993), p. 84.

16. Oriental and India Office Collection (OIOC), General Order of the Governor General, 21 September 1807, Bengal Military Consultations, 21 September 1807, P/22/35, no. 145. Cited in Douglas M. Peers, 'Soldiers, Surgeons and the Campaigns to Combat Sexually Transmitted Diseases in Colonial India, 1805–1860', *Medical History* 42, no. 2 (April 1998): 137–60.

17. OIOC, military letter from Bengal, 31 January 1824, F/4/835, no. 22, 253.

18. OIOC, lock hospital returns for 1828, Bengal Military Consultations, 31 July 1829, P/33/31 no. 81.

19. Kenneth Ballhatchet, *Race, Sex and Class under the Raj: Imperial Attitudes, and Policies and Their Critics, 1793–1905* (London: Weidenfeld and Nicolson, 1980), pp. 11–19.

20. Douglas M. Peers, 'War and Public Finance in Early Nineteenth-Century British India: The First Burma War', *International History Review* 11 (1989): 628–47. Cited in Peers, 'Soldiers, Surgeons and the Campaigns': 137–60, 151.

21. In the context of Victorian Britain, some of the famous works on the subject are as follows: P. McHugh, *Prostitution and Victorian Social Reform* (London: Croom Helm 1980); J.R. Walkowitz, *Prostitution and Victorian Society: Women, Class, and the State* (Cambridge: Cambridge University Press, 1982); Jeffrey Weeks, *Sex, Politics and Society: The Regulation of Sexuality since 1800*, 2nd edition (London: Pearson Education Ltd, 1989); Philippa Levine, 'Rough Usage: Prostitution, Law and the Social Historian', in *Rethinking Social History: English Society 1570–1920 and Its Interpretation*, edited by H.N. Wilson (Manchester: Manchester University Press, 1993); Paula Bartley, *Prostitution: Prevention and Reform in England, 1860–1914* (New York: Routledge, 2000).

22. R. Hyam, *Empire and Sexuality: The British Experience* (Manchester: Manchester University Press, 1990); Richard Phillips, 'Imperialism, Sexuality and Space: Purity Movements in the British Empire', in *Postcolonial Geographies*, edited by A. Blunt and C. McEwan (New York, London: Continuum, 2002).

23. Ann Laura Stoler, *Race and the Education of Desire: Foucault's History of Sexuality and the Colonial Order of Thing* (Durham, North Carolina, and London: Duke University Press, 1995).

24. The emergence of this mentality is explored in more depth in *The Facts of Life: The Creation of Sexual Knowledge in Britain, 1650–1950* by Roy Porter and Lesley Hall (New Haven: Yale University Press, 1995).

25. T.J. Wyke, 'Hospital Facilities for, and Diagnosis and Treatment of, Venereal Disease in England, 1800–1870', *The British Journal of Venereal Diseases* 49, nos 78–85 (1973): 81–2.

26. George Ballingall, who became professor of military surgery at the University of Edinburgh, surveyed surgeons in a number of stations and based on their reports, questioned the efficacy of mercury. He expounded on these views in several books, which were referred to as standard texts for surgeons in the army. George Ballingall, *Outlines of the Course of Lectures on Military Surgery, Delivered in the University of Edinburgh* (Edinburgh: Adam Black, 1833).

27. Michael Mason, *The Making of Victorian Sexuality* (Oxford: Oxford University Press, 1994), p. 58.

28. Sander L. Gilman, *Sexuality: An Illustrated History* (New York: Wiley, 1989), p. 238.

29. T.J. Wyke, 'The Manchester and Salford Lock Hospital, 1818–1917', *Medical History* 19 (1975): 73–86, 73.

30. This argument is developed in Mark Harrison, 'Tropical Medicine in Nineteenth-Century India', *Journal of History of Science* 25 (1992): 299–318. See also Mark Harrison, '"The Tender Frame of Man": Disease, Climate, and Racial Difference in India and the West Indies, 1760–1860', *Bulletin of History of Medicine* 70 (1996): 68–93.

31. John Clark, 'Report on Syphilis in H.M. Light Dragoons', *Madras Quarterly Medical Journal* 1 (1839): 370–410, 405. Cited in Peers, *Soldiers, Surgeons and the Campaigns*, p. 145.

32. Laura Briggs, *Reproducing Empire: Race, Sex, Science, and U.S. Imperialism in Puerto Rico* (California: University of California Press, 2002), p. 27.

33. An important new study of this relationship between sexuality and racism can be found in Stoler's, *Race and the Education of Desire*. Ashis Nandy also explores the question of how sexuality informed ideas and modes of power. He works with the premise that sexuality did not become complicit in colonial discourses until after 1830. (Ashis Nandy, *The Intimate Enemy: Loss and Recovery of Self under Colonialism* [New Delhi: Oxford University Press, 1983], pp. 5–6.)

34. Peers, *Soldiers, Surgeons and the Campaigns*, p. 138.

35. Captain Thomas Williamson, *East India Vade-Mecum*, vol. 2 (London: Black, Parry and Kingsbury, 1810), p. 423. Judy Whitehead in 'Bodies Clean and Unclean: Prostitution, Sanitary Legislation, and Respectable Femininity in Colonial North India', *Gender and History* 7, no. 1 (1995): 41–63, looks more

closely into how prostitutes fit into colonial constructions of Indian femininity. Cited in Peers, *Soldiers, Surgeons and the Campaigns*, p. 148.

36. Philippa Levine, 'Venereal Disease, Prostitution and the Politics of Empire: The Case of British India', *Journal of the History of Sexuality* 4 (1994): 579–602. Cited in Peers, *Soldiers, Surgeons and the Campaigns*, p. 149.

37. Kenneth MacKinnon, *A Treatise on Public Health, Climate, Hygiene and Prevailing Diseases of Bengal and the North-West Provinces* (Cawnpore: Cawnpore Press, 1848), p. 35. Cited in Peers, *Soldiers, Surgeons and the Campaign*, p. 149.

38. Levine, 'Venereal Disease, Prostitution, and the Politics of Empire': 585–6. Cited in Peers, *Soldiers, Surgeons and the Campaign*, p. 149.

39. OIOC, Report on the Lock Hospital Established at Bangalore, July 1855, Madras Military Consultations, 30 July–26 August 1856, P/273/41, no. 55. Cited in Peers, *Soldiers, Surgeons and the Campaign*, p. 149.

40. Clark, 'Report on Syphilis', p. 386. Cited in Peers, *Soldiers, Surgeons and the Campaign*, p. 149.

41. WIHM, Report on the Medical Topography and Statistics of the Presidency Division of the Madras Army, Madras, 1842, RAMC 2046. Cited in Peers, *Soldiers, Surgeons and the Campaign*, p. 155.

42. WIHM, John Hall, Medical Returns for 1851/52, RAMC 397/ERM1/2: 45. Cited in Peers, *Soldiers, Surgeons and the Campaign*, p. 155.

43. Among these are *The East India United Service Journal* (1833), *Transactions of the Medical and Physical Society of Calcutta* (1825 onwards), *Transactions of the Bombay Medical and Physical Society* (1838 onwards), and *Indian Journal of Medical and Physical Science* (1834 onwards). Essays on medical and military topics could also be found in the more general literature of the day, including the *Calcutta Review* (1844 onwards). For more information on the many medical societies which emerged in nineteenth-century India, see A. Neelameghan, *Development of Medical Societies and Medical Periodicals in India, 1780–1920* (Calcutta: Indian Association of Special Libraries and Information Centres, 1963). Cited in Peers, *Soldiers, Surgeons and the Campaign*, p. 156.

44. Edward M. Spiers, *The Army and the Society 1815–1914* (London: Longman, 1980), p. 135. Cited in Philippa Levine, 'Rereading the 1890s: Venereal Disease as "Constitutional Crisis" in Britain and British India', *Journal of Asian Studies* 55, no. 3 (August 1996): 585–612.

45. Frank Richards, *Old Soldier Sahib* (London: Faber and Faber, 1936); Waltraud Ernst, *Mad Tales from the Raj: The European Insane in British India 1800–1859* (London: Routledge, 1991), p. 15; Janaki Nair, *Women and Law in Colonial India: A Social History* (New Delhi and Bangalore: Kali for Women and National Law School of India University, 1996), p. 169. Cited in Levine, 'Rereading the 1890s': 589.

46. Arnold, *Colonizing the Body*, p. 85.

47. Cited in Ballhatchet, *Race, Sex and Class under the Raj*, p. 14.

48. Briggs, *Reproducing Empire*, p. 24.

49. Phillipa Levine, 'Orientalist Sociology and the Creation of Colonial Sexualities', *Feminist Review* 65 (Summer 2000): 5–21.

50. Ballhatchet, *Race, Sex and Class under the Raj*, p. 40.

51. Christopher Dandeker, *Surveillance, Power, and Modernity: Bureaucracy and Discipline from 1700 to the Present Day* (New York: St Martin's Press, 1990).

52. Michel Foucault, *Discipline and Punish: The Birth of the Prison* (London: Penguin Books, 1991), pp. 141–9.

53. See Stephen Legg, 'Governing Prostitution in Colonial Delhi: From Cantonment Regulations to International Hygiene (1864–1939)', *Social History* 34, no. 4 (November 2009): 447–67, 452.

54. Arnold, *Colonizing the Body*, p. 83.

55. Home Department, Public A, 20 February 1869, proceeding nos 112–15.

56. J.A. Crawford, Collector of Custom, to the Junior Secretary to the Board of Revenue, Lower Provinces, 30 September 1867, proceedings of the Home Department, Public A, 20 February 1869.

57. The British C.D. Act (1864) attempted to control venereal diseases by the compulsory medical examination of 'common prostitutes' in garrison towns and ten miles around. The Act was amended and extended in 1869. There is extensive literature available on the Contagious Diseases Acts, particularly on their origins in and impact on Britain itself. See, for example, F.B. Smith, 'Ethics and Disease in the Later Nineteenth Century: The Contagious Diseases Acts', *Historical Studies* 15 (1971): 118–35; F.B. Smith, 'The Contagious Diseases Acts Reconsidered', *Social History of Medicine* 3 (1990): 197–215; Walkowitz, *Prostitution and Victorian Society*; Paul Werth, 'Through the Prism of Prostitution: State, Society and Power', *Social History* 19, no. 1 (1994): 1–15.

58. J.A. Crawford, Collector of Custom, to the Junior Secretary to the Board of Revenue, Lower Provinces, 30 September 1869, proceedings of the Home Department, Public A, 20 February 1869.

59. C. Fabre-Tonnerre, Health Officer to Stuart Hogg, esquire, Chairman of the Justices of the Peace for the Town of Calcutta, 16 September 1867, Home Public Proceedings.

60. Despatch dated 16 September 1867 of C. Fabre-Tonnerre, Health Officer, to Stuart Hogg, esquire, Chairman of the Justices of the Peace for the Town of Calcutta, 16 September 1867, Home Public Proceedings, 1869. Cited in Sumanta Banerjee, 'The "Beshya" and the "Babu": Prostitute and Her

Clientele in 19th Century Bengal', *Economic and Political Weekly* 28, no. 45 (1993): 2461–72, 202n34.

61. Ashis Nandy, 'The Psychology of Colonialism: Sex, Age and Ideology in British India', *Psychiatry* 45 (1982): 197–218, especially 199.

62. *Report of the Sanitary Commissioner with the Government of India (SCGI)* (1867), p. 157; India Office Records (IOR), P/674. Government of India (GOI) (Sanitary), no. 204 (1871). Cited in Mark Harrison, *Public Health in British India: Anglo-Indian Preventive Medicine 1859–1914* (New Delhi: Cambridge University Press, Foundation Books, 1994), p. 89.

63. Home-Sanitary A, June 1875, nos 32–4.

64. Proceedings of the Lieutenant Governor of Bengal, General Department, 1874.

65. Proceedings of the Lieutenant Governor of Bengal, General Department, April, 1873.

66. Proceedings of the Lieutenant Governor of Bengal, General Department, April, 1873.

67. The annual report of the superintendent of lock hospitals on the working of the C.D. Act in Calcutta and its suburbs during the year 1881 pointed out (and the government, in its order of 25 May, admitted) that without such a power it was impossible to follow the Act effectively.

68. The Government of Bengal, file 1037, dated 30 August 1881, A, September, nos, 38–9.

69. Proceedings of the Government of Bengal, General Department, 1882.

70. Proceedings of Home-Sanitary Department, December 1884.

71. *Bengalee*, 21 August 1886, cited in Harrison, *Public Health in British India*, p. 75.

72. In 1869, Mrs Josephine Butler (1828–1906), with the support of Florence Nightingale, founded the Ladies National Association for the Repeal of the Contagious Diseases Acts on the grounds that they were unfair and one-sided, ignoring the role of men in the spread of the diseases. The Acts were suspended in 1883 and repealed in 1886.

73. Nandy, 'The Psychology of Colonialism'.

74. Levine, 'Venereal Disease, Prostitution, and the Politics of Empire'. Cited in Briggs, *Reproducing Empire*, p. 25n6.

75. Proceedings of the Lieutenant Governor of Bengal, General Department, April 1873.

76. OIOC, v/24/2292, Medical, 1877, Lock Hospitals, Resolution (17 July 1878), Darjeeling. Cited in Geraldine Forbes, *Women in Colonial India: Essays on Politics, Medicine, and Historiography* (New Delhi: Chronicle Books, an imprint of DC Publishers, 2005), p. 103n10.

77. Sujata Mukherjee, 'Imperialism, Medicine and Women's Health in Nineteenth Century India', in *Science and Society in India, c. 1750–2000*, edited by Arun Bandopadhyay (New Delhi: Manohar, 2010), pp. 95–120, 98.

78. Letter from A. Mackenzie Esq., C.S., Secretary to the Government of India, Home Department, to the Secretary to the Government of Bengal, 20 February 1883, Home-Sanitary, 1884, nos. 76–97.

79. Proceedings of the Lieutenant Governor of Bengal, General Department, April 1873. From S. Wauchope, Esq., C.B., Officiating Commissioner of Police, Calcutta, to the Secretary to the Government of Bengal, Judicial Department.

80. Briggs, *Reproducing Empire*, p. 27.

81. Whitehead, 'Bodies Clean and Unclean': 41. Cited in David Arnold, *The New Cambridge History of India*, vol. 3, part 5, *Science, Technology and Medicine in Colonial India* (Cambridge: Cambridge University Press, 2008), p. 90.

82. *Centenary Volume of Calcutta Medical College*, p. 124.

83. Sean Lang, 'Obstetrics and Obstruction: Maternity Provision in Madras, 1840–1852', in *From Western Medicine to Global Medicine: The Hospital Beyond the West*, edited by Mark Harrison, Margaret Jones, and Helen Sweet (New Delhi: Orient BlackSwan, 2009), pp. 108–41.

84. Harrison, Jones, and Sweet, *From Western Medicine to Global Medicine*, p. 17.

85. The CMC, which was established by the order of 20 February, ushered in a new era in the history of Western medicine in India. The CMC was the pioneer institution of the East for a systematic education in Western medicine. Its stated purpose was to train native youths aged between fourteen and twenty, irrespective of caste and creed, in the principles and practices of medical sciences in accordance with the mode adopted in Europe. Evidently, the purpose was to expand the reach of curative medicine accompanied by the growth of surgery, midwifery, and other medical practices.

86. Madras Public Consultations, 26 January 1841, no. 17, 272, OIOC P/247/58, 268, BL. Cited in Lang, 'Obstetrics and Obstruction', p. 113n23.

87. *Centenary Volume of Calcutta Medical College*, p. 23.

88. *Madras Public Consultations*, 26 January 1841, no. 17, 268, OIOC P/247/58,BL.Cited in Lang,'Obstetrics and Obstruction', p. 113n23.

89. *Centenary Volume of Calcutta Medical College*, p. 29.

90. *Centenary Volume of Calcutta Medical College*, Appendix III.

91. *Centenary Volume of Calcutta Medical College*, p. 31.

92. Proceedings of the Lieutenant Governor of Bengal, General (Medical) Department, April 1862.

93. Proceedings of the Lieutenant Governor of Bengal, General (Medical) Department, April 1862.

94. The number of European patients rose from 1,414 to 1,665, that of Eurasians from 7,741 to 8,211, that of Muslims decreased from 14,252 to 13,799, that of Hindus rose from 22,750 to 23,685, and others declined from 2,919 to 2,438. Proceedings of the Lieutenant Governor of Bengal, Home (Medical) Report of the Calcutta Medical Institutions, 1877.

95. Proceedings of the Lieutenant Governor of Bengal during June 1881. Medical and Municipal Department, Calcutta, 1881.

96. General Report on the Lunatic Asylums, Vaccination, and Dispensaries in the Bengal Presidency, 1868, p. 50, V/24/664, OIOC.

97. See Harrison, *Public Health in British India*, p. 90.

98. See *Centenary Volume of Calcutta Medical College*, p. 51. It was stated: 'Among 38 deaths out of 199 operations performed in 1879, the following causes of death were noted: Primary Haemorrhage-4; Secondary Haemorrhage-5; Tetanus-6; Erysepelas-5; Gangrene-4; Septicaemia-6; and Exhaustion-8.'

99. *Centenary Volume of Calcutta Medical College*, p. 52.

100. Joseph Lister introduced effective techniques for antisepsis. See Porter, *Cambridge History of Medicine*, p. 199.

101. *Centenary Volume of Calcutta Medical College*, p. 54.

102. *Centenary Volume of Calcutta Medical College*, p. 54.

103. *Centenary Volume of Calcutta Medical College*, p. 57.

104. Erwin Ackerknecht, *Medicine at the Paris Hospital 1794–1848* (Baltimore: Johns Hopkins University Press, 1967). Cited in David Armstrong, 'Bodies of Knowledge/Knowledge of Bodies', in *Reassessing Foucault: Power, Medicine and the Body*, edited by Colin Jones and Roy Porter (London and New York: Routledge, 1995), pp. 17–27.

105. See Armstrong, 'Bodies of Knowledge/Knowledge of Bodies', p. 19.

106. Armstrong, 'Bodies of Knowledge/Knowledge of Bodies', p. 19.

107. Armstrong, 'Bodies of Knowledge/Knowledge of Bodies', p. 20.

108. Michel Foucault, *The Birth of the Clinic: An Archaeology of Medical Perception* (London: Tavistock, 1973); Foucault, *Discipline and Punish*.

109. Michel Foucault, 'The Politics of Health in the Eighteenth Century', in *Power/Knowledge: Selected Interviews and Other Writings 1972–1977*, edited by Colin Gordon (New York: Pantheon Books, 1981), p. 166.

110. Foucault, *Birth of the Clinic*, p. vii.

111. Russell C. Maulitz, *Morbid Appearances: The Anatomy of Pathology in the Early Nineteenth Century* (Cambridge: Cambridge University Press, 1987). Cited in Mark Harrison, 'Racial Pathologies: Morbid Anatomy in British India, 1770–1850', in Harrison and Pati, *The Social History of Health and Medicine in Colonial India*, p. 175.

112. Harrison, 'Racial Pathologies'.

113. William Twinning, *Clinical Illustrations of the More Important Diseases of Bengal with the Results of an Enquiry into Their Pathology and Treatment*, 2nd edition (Calcutta: Mission Press, 1835), vol. 1, p. 27, vol. 2, pp. 437–8. Cited in Arnold, *Colonizing the Body*, p. 255. This clearly shows the importance attached to climate as well as topography in the tropical medicine of the late eighteenth and early nineteenth centuries, before the prevalence of the new paradigm of the germ theory of disease. See Arnold, *Colonizing the Body*, pp. 35–6.

114. Allen Web, *Pathologica Indica, or the Anatomy of Indian Diseases, based upon Morbid Specimens, from All Parts of the Indian Empire in the Museum of the Calcutta Medical College* (Calcutta: Thacker, 1848; first published 1843), p. 237. Cited in Harrison, 'Racial Pathologies', p. 186.

115. See Mel Gorman, 'Introduction of Western Science into Colonial India: Role of the Calcutta Medical College', *Proceedings of the American Philosophical Society* 132, no. 3 (September 1988): 276–98.

116. See Sujata Mukherjee, 'Women, Medicine and Empire: Female Practitioners and Patterns of Health Care in Colonial Bengal', *Historical Studies, Journal of the Department of History, Rabindra Bharati University* 2 (2001): 187–204.

117. Prankrishna Dutta, *Kolikatar Itibritto o Onyanyo Rachana* edited by Debasis Bose (Calcutta: Pustak Bipani, 1991), pp. 138–9.

118. Rosemary Fitzgerald, '"Making and Moulding the Nursing of the Indian Empire": Recasting Nurses in Colonial India', in *Rhetoric and Reality: Gender and the Colonial Experience in South Asia*, edited by Avril A. Powell and Siobhan Lambert-Hurley (New Delhi: Oxford University Press, 2006), pp. 185–222.

119. Harrison, Jones, and Helen Sweet, *From Western Medicine to Global*, p. 17.

2 *Medical Education and Emergence of Women Medics in Colonial Bengal*

A superstitious feeling is alleged to exist in the majority of Hindu families, principally cherished by the women and not discouraged by the men that a girl taught to read and write will soon after marriage become a widow. (W. Adam's Second Report on State of Education in Bengal, Rajshahi, 1836, reprinted in *One Teacher One School,* edited by Joseph Dibona [Delhi: Biblia Impex Pvt. Ltd, 1983], p. 91. Cited in Aparna Basu, 'A Century and a Half's Journey: Women's Education in India, 1850s to 2000', in *Women of India: Colonial and Post-Colonial Periods,* edited by Bharati Ray [New Delhi/Thousand Oaks/London: SAGE Publications, 2005], p. 183.)

I was born in the year 1814.... While I was a pupil in the Pathsala, at home I found my grandmother, mother and aunts reading books. They could write in Bengali and keep accounts. There were no female schools then. (Kalidas Nag, ed., *Bethune College and School, Centenary Volume, 1849–1949* [Calcutta: Saraswati Press, 1950], p. 2.)

> After some time the desire to learn how to read properly grew very strong in me. I was angry with myself for wanting to read books. Girls did not read.... People used to despise women of learning.... In fact older women used to show a great deal of displeasure if they saw a piece of paper in the hands of a woman. But somehow I could not accept this. (Rassundari Devi, 'Amar Jiban', in *Atmakatha*, vol. 1, edited by Nareshchandra Jana, Manu Jana, and Kamal Kumar Sanyal [Calcutta: Ananya Prakashan, 1981].)

Rassundari Devi, born in 1809, taught herself to read by stealing a few minutes from her housework and after taking care of twelve children. Rassundari overcame all opposition and obstacles, learnt to read and write, and penned her own experiences. The extract from her autobiography, presented at the beginning of the chapter, shows her passionate craving for knowledge. Apart from women's own desires, individual efforts of both Europeans and educated Indians, development of institutions, curricula, and official support were catalytic forces that helped the spread of female education in Bengal from the late nineteenth century; however, it was restricted mostly to the urban middle classes.

Surveys of indigenous education, undertaken by the governments of Bombay, Madras, and Bengal Presidencies in the 1820s and 1830s, recording an almost total absence of girl students from the village schools and from the Hindu and Muslim institutions of higher learning, lend credence to the first statement.[1] But it cannot be assumed that all women were illiterate. Females of aristocratic families were often given basic education, which would enable them to take care of property in case of the untimely demise of the husband.[2]

Many respectable Hindu families, like that of Pearychand Mitra (a great literary figure of Bengal in the nineteenth century), followed the practice of appointing Vaishnavis (women followers of the sixteenth-century Vaisnav saint Shri Chaitanya) to teach women at home. Sir Sayyid Ahmed Khan's mother, Azizunnisa Begum (1780–1857), a woman in strict purdah, knew Arabic and Persian.[3]

In nineteenth-century India, missionary efforts played a significant role in the spread of formal education for both men and women. The similarity between the spread of male and female education, however, ends there. The growth of education for women, in fact, followed an entirely different process as well as path than that of men. The motives for the promotion of education and patterns among the male population were completely different from those among women. State support for Western education, ushered in by Macaulay's Minute of 1835, had the political motive of creating loyal subjects of the Raj, while Indians welcomed the promotion of Western education since they viewed it as an instrument of progress and improvement. The Hindu bhadralok, or the urban, affluent elite—who gained economically by being associated with the new colonial economic structure imposed by the English East India Company's rule—showed eagerness to acquire and provide patronage to Western knowledge as it would become a key to socio-economic power as well as an instrument of indigenous social transformation.[4] As pointed out by Gyan Prakash, the 'cultural authority of science' and the authorization of the elite as agents of modernity and progress together attained 'an enduring dominance in India during the second half of the nineteenth century'.[5] Evidences show that even in the first half of the nineteenth century, indigenous reformers were eager to welcome Western science. The Hindu College, established through the efforts of the bhadraloks in Calcutta in 1817, had to teach—apart from the humanities—subjects like 'geography, chronology, astronomy, chemistry and other sciences'.[6] The college received a donation of scientific equipment from the British India Society of London for teaching astronomy, optics, mechanics, and chemistry in 1823.[7] In the same year, when the General Committee of Public Instruction (GCPI) decided to spend government funds to set up the Sanskrit College in Calcutta, Rammohan Roy, protesting against the decision, wrote to Lord Amherst:

> If it had been intended to keep the British nation in ignorance of real knowledge, the Baconian philosophy would not have been allowed to displace the system of schoolmen, which was the best calculated to perpetuate ignorance. In the same manner the Sanskrit system of education would be the best calculated to keep this country in darkness, if such had been the policy of the British Legislature.[8]

He urged the government to 'employ European gentlemen of talent and education to interest the natives of India in Mathematics, Natural Philosophy, Chemistry, Anatomy, and other useful sciences, which the natives of Europe have carried to a degree of perfection that has raised them above the inhabitants of other parts of the world'.

Opulent Calcuttans like Dwarakanath Tagore, Ramkamal Sen, and Motilal Seal were great patrons of Western medicine and philanthropists who generously contributed towards promoting medical education.[9] Statistics of the students collected at the end of the first ten years of the existence of the CMC showed that response from the Hindus and the Christian communities was good. Among the Hindus, the Brahmins, Kayasthas, Vaidyas, and weavers were particularly enthusiastic about medical education.

Social Reforms and Women's Education

Women's education was not motivated—at least initially—by an urge to create employment opportunities and facilitate women's entry into the professions or make them well acquainted with scientific learning. In fact, the aim, extent, and nature of female education remained a controversial subject for quite a long time. Sporadic attempts by some missionaries and Indian reformers for the spread of school education among girls in the 1820s and 1830s had very limited impact.[10] Formal female education in Bengal effectively took shape only after 1849, with the opening of the Bethune School.

During the second half of the nineteenth century, bhadralok reformers paid more attention to the education of middle-class women, which formed the core area in the agenda of reform of women's condition. Meredith Borthwick has argued that by 1860 social conditions became more favourable to the implementation of social reforms than before.[11] According to her, the influx of young men to Calcutta from the provinces of East Bengal gave rise to a group within the bhadralok community that was searching for a means of establishing its separate identity. She thus points out: 'In cooperation with members of established Calcutta *grihastha bhadralok* families, they provided a nucleus of people ready to adopt reform as a means of establishing their distinctiveness as a social group.'[12]

Apart from attempts of individual reformers (Radhakanto Deb, Ishwar Chandra Vidyasagar, and others) for upgrading women's condition, it was the Brahmo Samaj (founded as a religious organization by Rammohan Roy in 1828) as a group which provided support for the reform of women's conditions in Bengal. Issues like child marriage, widow remarriage, the breaking of purdah, and the education of women were all associated with one or another sect of the Brahmo Samaj.[13] After the first schism in the Brahmo Samaj in 1866, the Brahmo Samaj of India, led by reformer and religious leader Keshab Chandra Sen (the other sect was known as Adi Brahmo Samaj), became a staunch supporter of social reform more than ever. Keshab lectured on the importance of female education, and in 1863, male reformers organized a society, the Bamabodhini Sabha, for women's education. In the same year, Umesh Chandra Dutt started publishing the *Bamabodhini Patrika*, which carried articles on women's issues and organized an informal correspondence course for girls through its columns known as *antahpur siksha* or 'education in the seclusion of home'. The following decade witnessed serious debates and discussions amongst the Brahmo reformers regarding patterns of female education to be adopted. In fact, the Brahmo reformers became divided into two camps regarding the question of women's emancipation, including the question of patterns of education. In 1871, Keshab, who had at the time returned from a trip to England, became enthusiastic about women's education and started the Native Ladies' Normal School under the auspices of the Indian Reform Association. In his address on the occasion of the first anniversary of the Bama Hitaisini Sabha (a discussion group), Keshab pointed out that women should not aim at being great scholars, but at being good wives, mothers, daughters, and sisters. There was no need for women to learn 'manly' subjects such as geometry, philosophy, or natural science, he argued; instead, they should study domestic skills—housework and cooking—skills that would make them fit for their future work as wives and mothers. The students of the Native Ladies' Normal School were taken to public places such as the Asiatic Museum, but a separate time for viewing was arranged for them.[14] While the mainstream Brahmos like Keshab Sen and Umesh Chandra Dutt advocated limited education, all Brahmo reformers did not subscribe to Keshab's views. Thus the content of women's education became a contentious issue among the bhadralok class. Keshab's views were diametrically opposite to those of the radical Brahmos like Ananda Charan Khastagir, Dwarakanath Ganguly, Manmohan Ghosh, Durga Mohun Das, and Sivnath Sastri, who felt that both men and women should have equal opportunities in life. Radical Brahmos disagreed with Keshab Sen on the question as to why women should not sit together with men during Brahmo religious *sabhas* (assemblies). According to them, there was also no reason why there should be separate subjects for women or a limit to their achieving higher education, and they became vocal about providing the same opportunities for women in the field of education as was available to the male members of the society.

Progressive Brahmos, including Ananda Mohun Bose, Durga Mohun Das, and Sivnath Sastri, started the Samadarshi Party and a journal by the same name. The editor of the journal was Sivnath Sastri. Some reformers were deeply influenced by two British Unitarians—Mary Carpenter and Annette Akroyd. Mary Carpenter was the daughter of Rammohan Roy's Unitarian friend and associate, Lant Carpenter. One of her primary concerns was to break the monopoly of men in institutions of higher learning that awarded degrees. In fact, efforts to break male monopoly in higher education and extend equal opportunity to women were not restricted to Asia, but were a worldwide phenomenon in the nineteenth century. It was in 1878 that Oxford University established a college for women, the first degree-giving institution for women in the British Isles. Miss Annette Akroyd, who came to Calcutta in 1872, opened a school, the Hindu Mahila Bidyalaya, in November 1873, which aimed at spreading equal education for women.[15] After her wedding to Henry Beveridge in April 1875, the school ceased to operate and reopened later as the Banga Mahila Vidyalaya. Dwarakanath Ganguly, one of the radical Brahmos, became the headmaster while other progressive Brahmos (including Ananda Mohun Bose, Durga Mohun Das, and Sivnath Sastri) supported the move. Its first few students included daughters of eminent Brahmos such as Durga Mohun Das' daughters, Sarala and Abala, Jagadish Chandra Bose's sister, Swarnaprabha, Manmohan Ghosh's sister, Binodini, and also Kadambini Basu, daughter of Brajakishore Basu.

On 1 August 1878, this school was merged with the Bethune School to become Bethune College. The progressive members of the Sadharan Brahmo Samaj, who had left Keshab's Brahmo Samaj of India to form their own *samaj* (society) in 1878, petitioned the government to affiliate Bethune College with Calcutta University. After affiliation, Kadambini Basu, a Brahmo, and Chandramukhi Basu, a Christian, became the first recipients of the B.A. degree from Bethune College in 1882, becoming the first women graduates in the entire British empire.[16]

Women's Medical Education: Indian Support and Colonial Policy

Brahmo reformers like Durga Mohun Das and Dwarakanath Ganguly were enthusiastic supporters of medical education for women.[17] It was as early as 1875 that a member of the Brahmo community, Neel Kamal Mitra, petitioned to have his granddaughter, Biraj, admitted to the Hospital Assistant course at the CMC. Mitra insisted that there should be separate sitting arrangement for her granddaughter and also that her husband should be allowed to accompany her to the dissection room. Ultimately, nothing came out of this proposal.[18]

The growth of public opinion in favour of women's medical education also became visible when a number of newspapers and journals emphasized the need for women doctors trained in Western medicine for women patients. The imperative of getting female doctors to spread health care among reclusive women patients, who were not receiving proper treatment because of social conservatism, made it somewhat easy to find a moral consensus on the introduction of women's medical education. One prevalent practice in Hindu society, which seemed to obstruct delivery of proper medical care to women, was that of avoidance of any contact between women patients and doctors. The indirect method of treating women patients by male doctors was narrated by Koilash Chunder Bose, assistant surgeon, who testified in the Bose versus Bose adultery case (1878) thus:

> The custom for Hindu ladies is to instruct others [male members] about their ailments. The rule is to communicate through a maidservant, her mother, or guardian. It did not strike me at all as strange that Upendro should instruct me. The disease is very common among women…I never spoke to Khettermoney, about that sort of thing. I did not treat her. I asked her about it through the maidservant and she denied.[19]

The *Brahmo Public Opinion*, which favoured women's medical education, wrote:

> We know of several instances in orthodox Hindu families, where the female members suffer from the most complicated diseases, but yet would not allow male doctors to visit and treat them. The consequence is, they are treated second-hand through the assistance of uneducated quack

> native midwives, and in ninety-nine out of a hundred, they are never radically cured.[20]

For the Indian reformers (just as for the colonizers), Indian women's disinclination to male doctors was the basis of an argument in favour of the proposal to train female doctors. The admission of women into medical education meant an acceptance that women would be employed as doctors, or would practise as doctors. In fact, the logic of gender segregation paved the way for a strong argument in favour of women service providers, not only in health care but also in a few other professions such as teaching. At the same time, it cannot be forgotten that many Indian reformers—particularly those arguing for women's equal opportunities in education—were convinced about the usefulness of scientific education. For example, Dwarakanath Ganguly, a radical Brahmo and the teacher, mentor, and husband of Kadambini, pointed out in 1879: 'Rather than learning the fine geographic details of various countries, it would be worthwhile to examine whether or not it is more relevant to have a basic knowledge of Physiology.'[21]

In the field of women's medical education, however, Bengal did not provide the leadership. Madras played the pioneering role in this regard. In 1875, a new chapter in the history of medical education opened when four female students—all of European or Anglo-Indian origin—entered the premises of Madras Medical College as students of the three-year certificate class. At that time, there was no choice but to induct women into the general medical colleges, where instructions were given by male teachers and attended by male students. It is noteworthy that the initiative in Madras was taken well ahead of many European countries, where the debate about women's medical education raged in various cities. The London School of Medicine for Women, in fact, was established the same year that Madras admitted women to its medical institution. The credit for introducing medical education to women goes to a doctor, a government official, and also to Mary Scharlieb, wife of an English barrister in Madras (later to become a London gynaecologist).[22] Mary Scharlieb came to India in 1866 and took a one-year course in midwifery at the Madras Maternity Hospital but found the training inadequate to meet all the needs. For getting formal training in medical science, she approached the then governor of Madras, Lord Hobart, and Dr Balfour, surgeon general, to grant her permission to join the Madras Medical College. However, Dr Balfour, a firm supporter of this proposal, failed to convince the Director of Public Instruction (DPI), who considered it to be 'entirely premature'. Despite this, Dr Balfour persisted with his recommendation, and finally, with the support of Dr Furnell—the principal of Madras Medical College—obtained the required permission.

In Bombay, the Medical Women's Fund was set up in 1882 by George A. Kittredge, an American businessman, to raise public subscription for the promotion of female medical education. Kittredge was helped in his endeavour by a rich Parsee, Sorabji Shapurji Bengali, and was able to collect Rs 40,000 within two months. The effort gained further momentum when Pestonji Hormusji Kama came forward to offer a donation of Rs 1,64,300. From outside India, British women themselves showed a great deal of concern for providing medical care to Indian female patients by encouraging the growth of women's medical professions. Dr Frances Elizabeth Hoggan (one of the first British women to qualify as a doctor) thought that the Indian Medical Service (IMS) had failed to cater to the medical requirements of Indian women, and that only women doctors could best serve the interests of Indian female patients.[23] She pointed out that the 'shrinking' of women patients from male doctors was not a 'prejudice' to be disregarded but a 'natural' attitude, and it was the 'right of Indian women' to expect this sentiment to be 'respected and not outraged'. In a meeting of the National Indian Association held at Cavendish Square, Bombay, in November 1882, Dr (Mrs) Frances Hoggan read a paper on 'Medical Women in India' and urged that what was needed was a new medical department for women working in harmony with the existing Civil Medical Service. She suggested that the government should produce two classes of medical women: (*a*) ordinary practitioners who would provide health care in the countryside, and (*b*) the other more accomplished group who would be capable of acting as teachers as well as practitioners in the bigger towns.[24]

Mrs Garret Anderson, MD, expressed the opinion that Indian females themselves should be prepared to help themselves as their needs were too enormous to be taken care of by a small number of English lady doctors. According to her, very few English ladies were ready to come to India if there was no chance of making a larger income than they could get in England. In 1883, the Kitteridge Fund applied to the

Bombay University to allow the admission of women into medical classes and degrees. A certificate class was opened for non-matriculate students. The Cama hospital set up in 1886 had three successive women superintendents, Dr Edith Pechey, Dr Annette Benson, and Dr Eliza Turner Watts, who worked diligently and played, besides treating the sick, a leading role in educating and training women doctors.

Bengal was far ahead than the other two presidencies in the matter of female education since it produced the first ever female graduates in British India. In the case of medical education, around 1876, Lieutenant Governor Sir Richard Temple expressed support of the demand for the admission of female students to CMC classes. In 1879, the matter was again discussed; but on neither occasion did the discussion have any practical result.[25]

In a letter addressed to the principal of CMC, dated 5 May 1882, A.W. Croft, DPI, wrote: 'The parents of two or three young ladies, European and native, who have passed the Entrance Exam of the University, have expressed to me their strong desire that their daughters should join the medical College.'[26]

In January 1882, Ellen Barbara d'Abreu (born in Dhaka to an Anglo-Indian family from Patna and Nagpur) and Abala Das (daughter of the renowned Brahmo reformer Durga Mohun Das, who later married the scientist Jagadish Chandra Bose) passed the First Arts and Entrance Examinations respectively, from the Bethune School. D'Abreu and Das approached A.W. Croft in Bengal to get admission at CMC. In May 1882, Mr Croft asked for the opinion of the principal and the council of the Medical College regarding the possibility of the admission of females to the CMC classes. He urged that they should be admitted on the grounds that this would probably result in great alleviation of suffering if there were a body of qualified practitioners who could be admitted to zenanas without any objection, as well as on the grounds that if the Medical College classes were thrown open to females, a career of usefulness would be provided for those ladies who were passing the university examinations. According to Croft, 'conditions of social life in this country, required a body of thoroughly trained and qualified female practitioners' in order to rescue 'large numbers of the women of India, either from a life of suffering or from premature death'.[27]

Mr Croft proposed to recommend to the university the admission of female candidates if they passed the Entrance examination. Mr Croft's suggestion was laid before the council of the CMC, and at a meeting of the council at which five members were present, resolutions were passed by a majority of four adverse to the proposition. It was pointed out that no general demand for female physicians existed amongst the native community. The council members did not hesitate to express the opinion that 'extended training in midwifery and diseases of women and children will suffice to meet the requirements of the case'. The two applicants then moved to the Medical College of Madras. D'Abreu entered the BM class (five years) and Abala Das the LMS class (four years). These two students were later granted scholarships by the DPI.[28]

The majority in the council of the CMC also thought that 'mixed classes' of men and women were 'objectionable' and 'likely to exercise a demoralizing influence upon students of both sexes',[29] and that separate schools had to be provided if women were to be trained in medicine. On one point, that of lowering the qualification for entrance to the CMC, the whole council was unanimously adverse.[30]

Dr Coats, principal of the CMC, was one of the most liberal advocates of women's admission into medical classes. He quoted authorities in Switzerland and France who believed that the presence of women in medical classes had a 'refining influence'.[31] Dr Harvey, professor of midwifery, was also a strong advocate of women's medical education. As the teacher of midwifery, he was the only member of the council with experience of lecturing to mixed classes, and argued in favour of such teaching arrangements. To strengthen his case, he pointed out that he had not experienced any unbecoming incident or behaviour on the part of the male students. Fortunately, not only the principal and the DPI but also the lieutenant governor of Bengal, Rivers Thompson, were sympathetic to the cause of female medical education. The lieutenant governor felt that Bengal's reputation as a leader in educational progress in British India was at stake since Madras and Bombay had already begun to admit women to medical classes and Bengal was lagging behind. It was unacceptable, he mentioned, that Bengal, a progressive province in other respects, should be illiberal and retrograde in this. It should not lag behind in providing medical education to ladies, especially since it was not 'the prejudices of native parents' that was the problem. He argued that 'legitimate private interests' were being hindered by the attitude which the Medical College council assumed. The lieutenant governor also pointed out that the members of the council, in denying women entry into medical education, were encouraging social conservatism, and therefore zenana prejudices. He was not willing to stifle 'the natural and reasonable aspirations of Indian ladies to enter a profession which would find in India, of all countries in the world, a wide sphere of action and of beneficent service'. It was subsequently decided by the lieutenant governor in 1883 that women should be admitted to the classes in the CMC on the same footing as male students.[32] Separate admission criteria for women, even though it was shown to be prevalent in other parts of India, were not accepted in Bengal.[33] The lieutenant governor would open the college doors wide to students of both sexes, but he would not specially favour either sex because of two reasons: first, liberal training and training in powers of observations were especially required in the medical profession and second, it would be conferring a 'fatal gift' on the cause of women's medical education to start them off on a weaker foot.[34] He dismissed the opposition with the hope that he could count on the loyalty and zeal of the professors to bring his policy on this question to a successful issue, despite their objections.[35]

During debates regarding women's admission to CMC, the policymakers' stated objective was, at least partially, to bring about good governance delivering public good. According to the lieutenant governor, the fact that 'some Bengali ladies, fully qualified by educational attainments' had to go to 'the more liberal Presidency of Madras' to study medicine was 'clearly opposed to the public good'.[36]

The policymakers were convinced that Indian women were generally averse to being treated by male doctors. This formed the powerful basis of an argument in favour of the proposal to train female doctors. The lieutenant governor also opined that 'the misery caused by neglected and unskillfully treated illness' was widespread and 'most lamentable'. He also accepted the view that Indian women 'in every position of life' would prefer death to treatment by a male physician. The only solution to these problems seemed to be to extend medical education to women.[37]

Moreover, he dismissed the objection raised on the ground of teaching mixed classes as obsolete and cited experiences of Europe and America and even of India, that is, Madras, which had in fact shown that mixed classes could be taught without adverse results. In Madras, there was no sign of demoralization due to mixed classes.[38] Female entry into medical profession, however, was not welcomed by all. Some of the contemporary journals and anonymous letters to the editors of these journals criticized the government for having acted in haste, without scrutinizing the matter intensively as what was being experimented with were precious human lives. The decision to facilitate women's entry into the medical profession was even frowned upon in IMS circles. The *IMG* attacked the government in its editorials time and again. Over the beginning in Madras, it had rebuked the policymakers sarcastically that the demand for female doctors by the people of India was a pure assumption to start with; that females of any kind were fit to be doctors was indeed questionable in India; and the manner in which it was being carried out was superficial and unsafe. Another editorial of the same journal expressed its view in 1884 that women were better fitted for nursing than being doctors, and that an agency of educated nurses would fulfil the requirements of the country better than one of full-fledged lady doctors. Perhaps, jealousy and fear of competition in a hitherto all-male profession generated such fierce opposition and derogatory comments. The first female medical students had to face and overcome even more serious charges of moral turpitude. The superintendent of the Temple Medical School, Patna, reported in 1895 that anonymous petitions were frequently received which denounced the morals of the female students. That was due to the want of a hostel or dwelling house for them, as he pointed out that 'at present they had to live in the bazaar, and unless they were living with relatives, that was a most undesirable arrangement'. Despite all these social discriminations and discouragement, female medical education, continued to spread and flourish. The first beneficiary of the new rule was Kadambini Basu, one of the first female graduates in India, who later married the Brahmo reformer Dwarakanath Ganguly. To facilitate women's entry into the medical college, a scholarship of Rs 20 per month was provided to all female medical students without restriction of number for a period of five years. Kadambini received this scholarship with provision for retrospective effect from July 1883. In 1884, A.W. Croft extended the scholarships of Ellen d'Abreu and Abala Das to continue their study at the Medical College of Madras since they had moved prior to the opening of classes to women in Calcutta.[39] His argument was that the medical education of these women would benefit Bengal when they returned. Croft also granted these scholarships to two notable students—Virginia Mary Mitter (Nandy) (1856–1945) and Bidhumukhi Bose (daughter of Bhuban Mohan Bose, a Bengali-speaking Christian from Dehradun; sister of Chandramukhi Bose)—after receiving their applications for scholarships to study at the CMC. Miss Virginia Mitter was later to prove wrong the anticipated fears of undesirability of the mixed classes and lowering of the educational standards when she headed the list of successful candidates in 1888.

In 1885, Maharani Swarnamayi of Cossim Bazar granted one and a half lakh rupees to build a hostel for female students at the CMC, which 'removed a great obstacle in the way of female students studying medicine in Calcutta'.[40] The Nawab Begum of Murshidabad donated Rs 25,000 for the erection of a hostel for the female students of Campbell Medical School, Sealdah, which was to be named at her insistence as 'Lady Elliot Hostel'. The balance of the estimated expenditure of Rs 96,000 was to come from a bequest of Rs 90,000 left by the late Walter Thomson of Beheea in 1892 at the disposal of the lieutenant governor for promoting scientific and secular education of women in Bengal. Moreover, the district and municipal boards showed commendable attempts at creating special scholarships for female students in the vernacular-medium schools of their respective areas.

The Campbell Medical School was originally established in 1872 to accommodate the rising number of applicants who wished to enrol in the Bengali programme of the CMC, started in 1853. The 1880s witnessed increasing enthusiasm among women students for entry into the programme of vernacular medical education. In 1887, Sir A.W. Croft wrote to the secretary of Bengal:

> I have the honour to state that I have been lately in communication with the Superintendent of the Campbell Medical School on the subject of establishing in that institution a vernacular medical class for female students, to be taught the same course, during the same period of three years, as the male students who now read in that institution. Dr. Coull Mackenzie expresses his entire concurrence in the proposal. He admitted that it was impossible to say, without a trial, whether the classes would be popular and well attended. He also mentioned that ever since the

> movement for the medical education of women in India began, he had in mind the formation of a school of this kind, and hoped that it would be successful.

Croft also pointed out that his original idea was that the medical education of women in this country should be divided into three grades: first, the English course at the Medical College for the degree or the license in medicine; second, the purely vernacular classes; and third, classes for the instruction of midwives. The first and third were running successfully, the second was substituted with the certificate class at the Medical College in which instruction was imparted in English because the professors of the College were unable to teach in the vernacular. He mentioned that this class was practically confined to young European and Eurasian women, who would only practise in the large towns. It in no way met his desire for the creation of a class of medical women for the larger villages of the mofussil, practising under the same conditions and among the same class of people as the young men trained in the vernacular medical schools of Calcutta, Dhaka, Patna, and Cuttack. He further wrote:

> That is the object of my present proposal; and though I am fully aware that it is by no means certain to succeed owing to the general (though I am glad to say diminishing) want of education among women throughout Bengal, and to the obstacles which social conditions impose to their prosecution of an independent career, yet I am of opinion that the practical benefits that would follow from such a measure, if happily it should be successful, justify Govt. in making the experiment. If it succeeds, well and good; if it fails, little or no cost is incurred and no harm is done.[41]

J.M. Coats, the principal of CMC, claimed that numerous district boards informed him about their requirements to employ female medical practitioners whom they could pay around Rs 30–40 per month. They were unable to afford recruiting graduates of CMC who generally expected a minimum salary of Rs 300 per month. It seemed that there were also eager applicants who wanted to get enrolled in the vernacular programme, if offered an opportunity. According to Dr S.C. Mackenzie, the superintendent of Campbell Medical School, right at that moment fifteen candidates were available who included 'ladies belonging to the most respectable *brahmo* families of Bengal—one of them is a relative of a pleader, another—a relative of a Government inspector of schools, another—a relative of the superintendent of a Zoological Garden, and two others are relatives of a teacher of a medical school'.[42] Not unlike what happened in the case of the CMC, there were some who opposed this move of admitting female students at Campbell. Surgeon Major C.J.W. Meadows, officiating civil surgeon of Patna, wrote to the secretary to the Government of Bengal: 'I am…of opinion that no special demand or need exists for this inferior class of Female Hospital Assistants in the villages, and their employment would tend rather to discredit the Western system of medicine and so defeat the object in view.'[43] His view was supported by R.L. Dutt, officiating civil surgeon of Rungpore. According to the latter, there was no need for medical women of the hospital assistant class in mofussils. He also suggested that Indian women who wanted to become doctors should attend medical college and those with less education should take the midwifery course.[44] Some even pointed out that Indian women were too steeped in ignorance and tradition to want Western medical care.[45]

Eventually, however, all obstacles were overcome, and in 1888, the Campbell Medical School at Sealdah finally opened its door to female students. The first batch of fifteen female trainees admitted at Campbell included Hindus, Brahmos, native Christians, and Eurasians. Unlike the CMC, Campbell's instructors were Indians who received their medical training in India. Textbooks were written either in Bengali or were translations of English books. Different scholarship schemes were introduced by the Dufferin Fund from 1885 onwards.

The British considered themselves to be the 'enlightened outsiders' whose moral responsibility lay in upgrading the colonized. From the point of view of the colonizers, the imperative of women doctors was articulated as part of the 'white man's burden'.[46] Western opinion was also thus largely convinced that only female agents could hope to make metropolitan medical care more palatable to Indian women. Several scholars have pointed out, quite rightly, that compared to England, women in India entered medical colleges and the medical profession quite easily.[47] Yet, progress of education was rather slow—most upper-class and upper-caste Muslim and Hindu women were not able to leave the seclusion of the home to become medical students. Patriarchal social norms ensured that, at least during the initial days of female medical education, very few Hindu and Muslim females joined the profession. According to the Calcutta Census of 1901, 124 women were registered as qualified medical practitioners.[48] According to one estimate of 1907, 17 students out of a total of 425 students studying at the CMC were female.[49]

In 1912, medical colleges all over India had female students mainly from the European, Eurasian, and Indian Christian communities. There were very few Hindus.[50] In Campbell, in the first two years (1888–90), there were more Hindu women, mostly Brahmins and Kayasthas. In 1890, there were eight Brahmos, eight Christians, and twelve Hindu women entrants. Hindu girls included, apart from Brahmins and Kayasthas, one Vaidya and one Vaisnav.[51] In 1891, the first Muslim woman was admitted, followed by the second one in 1893. Around 1893–4, out of a total of thirty-one female students, three were Europeans, seven Hindus, seven Brahmos, two Muslims, and ten native Christians. From 1890, all candidates were required to pass a special elementary examination in English. After 1896, it became a four-year programme. Examinations became more difficult and a greater understanding of English was required. According to Geraldine Forbes, the number of Bengali women among the student community began to decline gradually after 1896 due to stringent admission rules. More native Christian, European, and Eurasian women entered the school.[52] Outside Calcutta, the Dacca Medical School also admitted female students. Their number was, however, very small. During 1916–17 there were two students. Next year the number rose to seven and to ten in 1919–20.[53] Women medical students disproportionately consisted of women belonging to European, Eurasian, and Indian Christian communities, which placed fewer restrictions on the employment and education of women. Wherever Hindu and Muslim females appeared, they were very few in number. This pattern continued until the 1930s.[54] Between 1935 and 1940, however, the number of Anglo-Indian students declined while the number of Hindu and Muslim students started to rise.

Racialism and Gender Discrimination

British racism ensured that medical education in colonial India developed on a tiered basis: Indian men were relegated to the lower ranks as 'hospital assistants', while Europeans and Eurasians received 'licentiate of medicine and surgery' or 'assistant surgeons' degrees. Indian women, too, were clustered among the 'hospital assistant' or 'certificate' ranks. The official view explicitly stated that hospital assistants were supposed to supply cheap medical aid to the country districts but were 'not intended to take charge or to be placed on an equal footing with ladies possessing superior qualifications.'[55]

The introduction of medical training for women in institutions like CMC and Campbell Medical School created different categories of qualified female medical professionals, just as it did among the male trainees. Among women who received training at CMC were many who belonged to enlightened, educated families. After 1885, many zenana hospitals were established by the contributions made by the Dufferin Fund, a philanthropic organization which was started in 1885, or the National Association for Supplying Female Medical Aid to Indian Women. Dufferin hospitals and dispensaries, opened after 1885 with private donations and government support, provided employment to many women doctors.[56] According to the 1904 report of the Bengal branch of the Dufferin Fund, thirty-eight of the Fund's forty-three female hospitals and dispensaries were under women hospital assistants who were Vernacular Licentiate in Medicine and Surgery (VLMS) degree holders. The majority of them were graduates of Campbell Medical School.[57]

Various hospitals which facilitated Indian women's entry into the medical profession also practised racial discrimination. Appointments were given to white doctors even when more efficient Indian female doctors were available. Posts opened up by the Lady Dufferin Fund, which had been set up to bring medical treatment to the zenana women of India, were monopolized by Europeans and Eurasians. In fact, in 1905, there were complaints that the European lady superintendent of the Dufferin Hospital in Calcutta was dismissing native nurses in favour of European nurses from Bombay. The Dufferin Fund was, in fact, criticized by a section of the Indian elite because the onus of financial responsibility fell in large part on the Indians for a cause which seemed to serve better the interest of the British imperialists rather than the Indians. It was strongly apprehended that the real beneficiaries of the Fund would be European rather than Indian female doctors. In Britain, sexual discrimination against women limited their career opportunities as male doctors specializing in obstetrics and gynaecology tried to restrict the number of female competitors in the field. The general prevalent attitude, that women were fit only to treat women patients, further limited job opportunities for women physicians. In such a situation, the Dufferin Fund provided a very convenient outlet for qualified British lady doctors who were willing to take up jobs in India. Discrimination against women doctors in England forced them to look to the colonies for employment. In India, English women doctors were able to take advantage of racial discrimination of the colonial power to monopolize all available positions, thereby hindering the advancement of Indian women doctors. As pointed out by scholars, Indian women were disadvantaged in a system 'that placed men above women, foreign credentials above those earned in India, and discounted knowledge of local languages and customs.'[58] The vernacular press voiced strong objections to the discriminatory policies of the colonial government and criticized the practice of spending great amounts of public revenue on hiring European lady doctors who did not speak vernacular languages when qualified Bengali lady doctors were available in increasing numbers. European lady doctors also charged higher fees.

Biographical evidence shows how far and in what ways the racism and sexist outlook prevailing in society hindered the professional career and personal life of women doctors. Kadambini Basu, the daughter of Brahmo reformer Braja Kishore Basu, who entered the CMC in 1883, received the Graduate of Bengal Medical College (GBMC) degree in 1886 instead of the MB degree because she failed in one part of her final practical examinations.[59] Professor R.C. Chandra failed her in medicine. It was generally believed to have been a vindictive gesture because he was opposed to the inclusion of women in the CMC. In 1888, Kadambini was appointed doctor at the Lady Dufferin Women's Hospital in Calcutta and received a monthly salary of Rs 300. She, however, was not granted a permanent post in 1891. *The Bengalee* pointed out that high positions in the Dufferin Fund hospitals were reserved for European and Eurasian women and cited Kadambini's credentials, a B.A. and a GBMC, as superior to those of any other candidate, including the woman hired for the job. It also remarked that none of the employees of the Bengal Dufferin Fund had any degree, medical or otherwise.[60] Kadambini argued that exclusion of Indian women from the best hospital jobs prevented them from developing their skills. They would miss all the advantages of such professional duties due to their exclusion from the medical charge of important hospitals, or by being placed in an inferior position there, for in the inferior class of hospitals, few cases of importance would ever go for treatment. At the large and important hospitals, the major operations and other important duties were always likely to be performed by senior persons in charge.

Kadambini set up a successful private practice. Her patients included women of the Nepalese royal family. In 1893, she was sent to Edinburgh for higher studies. She had to face humiliation when a section of the conservative Hindu society launched a slander campaign against her. 'In 1891, *Bangabasi* (Resident of Bengal), a journal of the Hindu orthodoxy, accused Kadambini of being a fitting—and therefore despicable—example of a modern Brahmo woman. Though by then Kadambini was a mother of five, and a responsible housewife, the author of this article accused her of being a whore.'[61]

Her husband, Dwarakanath Ganguly, and other Brahmo friends including Sivnath Sastri and Nilratan Sarkar started legal action against the journal and its editor. The editor, Mahesh Chandra Pal, was found guilty. He was fined Rs 100 and was sentenced to six months' imprisonment. By established conservative norms of thought in Hindu society, maintenance of female virtues was incompatible with social liberty. The male members were not ready to allow social mobility to women because they feared that it would slacken their control and domination over female members. Kadambini was, however, a courageous and independent lady and was fortunate to have the support of her husband and other progressive Brahmos. Other women were not so fortunate. Virginia Mary Mitter, for example, assisted her husband Dr Purnachandra Nandi but never practised independently. Jamini Sen—who remained unmarried—on the other hand, pursued a long and successful career. She belonged to an educated Brahmo family. She was the daughter of Chandicharan Sen, who was a sub-judge, and sister of poet Kamini Roy. She joined the CMC in 1890 and won distinction in the fourth year, receiving a first in Materia Medica. In 1912, she received the Diploma of the Royal Faculty of Physician and Surgeon, Glasgow.

Women students of Campbell Medical School who received the VLMS degree and found employment as hospital assistants in district hospitals, also often became victims of the racist and sexist outlook. The autobiography of Dr Haimabati Sen, a Campbell graduate, records her experiences as a student and professional doctor and gives us a glimpse into the hardships and struggle she faced in her personal and professional life.[62]

Haimabati Sen was born in Khulna district of eastern Bengal (now in Bangladesh) in 1866. Her father was a wealthy zamindar who allowed her to spend her days in the outer quarters and also receive education. Her mother and grandmother—very much against her father's wishes—arranged her marriage when she was only nine and a half to an affluent, forty-five-year-old kulin kayastha husband—twice widowed, with two daughters nearly of her age (kayasthas are among the upper castes in the Hindu caste hierarchy among the Bengalis and 'kulin kayastha' signified a distinctive group among the kayasthas). She became a widow within a year. After the death of her parents and mother-in-law, she was ill-treated by her brother-in-law and went to Benares and became a teacher at a small school for girls. Hearing about Brahmo Samaj institutions to educate widows, Haimabati came to Calcutta. She met Brahmo leaders and remarried a Brahmo Samaj worker, Kunjabehari. The marriage turned out to be a difficult one for Haimabati. There was no steady income, and even after five children (four sons and one daughter) had been born, her husband remained unmindful about his responsibilities.

Haimabati joined the Campbell Medical School in 1891 at the age of twenty-six, along with a few other girls. She received a scholarship of Rs 8 per month from the government, plus school fees. At the end of the first year, she was placed first in the examination and was awarded two scholarships. Later, when the final examinations took place, she topped the class, scoring more than all the male students. The boys in her college immediately went on strike in protest against her being awarded the gold medal. Ultimately she gave up the gold and accepted a silver medal.

She had a brilliant academic career, but finding a job was not easy, disadvantaged as she was by race and gender exploitation. Haimabati joined the Hooghly Lady Dufferin Women's Hospital, Chinsurah, as a lady doctor in 1894. Her salary was Rs 40 per month, and later it became Rs 50. With the job also came free living quarters, and alongside, she was allowed to have a private medical practice.

Haimabati endured constant hardships in her professional as well as personal life. She was placed under the supervision of the assistant surgeon and the civil surgeon. Her memoir tells us that she was sexually harassed and physically assaulted. The assistant surgeon, Dr Badrikanath Mukherjee attempted to seduce her and even sent goondas to beat her up. When she complained, the civil surgeon rebuked her for being arrogant.

While Dr Mukherjee harassed her, the civil surgeons controlled her professional life. They were appointed supervisors of the Dufferin Hospital and called 'Boss' by her. Most of them maltreated her, although one of them treated her kindly. She also took up private practice and supported her family with her income. Haimabati had eight pregnancies and five children. She died of breast cancer in 1933.

Haimabati's life was very unusual and unconventional. She accepted salaried posts (as teacher and then as a lady doctor) when it was not really socially acceptable. In all her jobs, she became the object of sexual harassment. She also had to attend to her duties as a housewife and mother. Her memoir tells us a lot about violence against women in colonial India. She fought back against all her attackers except for her husband. It seems that she accepted male domination and domestic violence within her own marriage. She painted her husband vividly as a man who did not contribute financially for the family or to raise the children and used her money. He also made all decisions and sometimes abused her. But apparently she obeyed her husband.

Many less prominent lady doctors who took up practices in the mofussils were often subjected to hostile and derisive reactions from the local male population. The 'Malda Lady Doctors' case' of 1902 has been considered as an extreme example of male contempt for women doctors.[63] Pramilabala, a lady doctor belonging to Malda, was called out at night on the false pretext of attending the wife of the zamindar Madan Gopal Chaudhuri, and taken to his boat and assaulted. She charged Chaudhuri of abduction with evil intent, and 'of having used criminal force with intent to outrage her modesty'. A fine of Rs 1,000 was imposed on the accused. Newspaper reports, however, expressed indignation at the light punishment inflicted.[64]

Impact

No doubt, hostility and occasional aggression made it extremely difficult for female doctors to carry out their professional duties. On the positive side, the opening of medical education for women doctors created new opportunities, and a section of urban reformist Bengalis were able to utilize this opportunity for self-improvement. Women who became doctors gained professional prestige and were rewarded with the possibility of earning a substantial independent livelihood. A sound foundation for female medical education and their legitimate place in the medical establishment of the country was laid during these struggling years, on which women of the coming generations built successful careers. Those who received new medical education gained an occupational or professional identity which was enmeshed with their gender identity (see Appendix 2A for some evidence of qualified women physicians who found different employments).

The presence of women practitioners in the districts made Western medicine available to a significant number of women who could now be treated in their homes or hospitals and dispensaries. Women patients were offered more options of choosing from different kinds of practitioners, including qualified male and female practitioners of Western, as well as indigenous, medicine.

The struggle of women doctors also exposed the policy of racial discrimination practised by colonizers and the sexist outlook prevailing in society. No doubt, it threw a challenge to patriarchal domination and subordination, and prepared the background for demanding better and equal opportunities for health care to women. The growth of medical education and entry of women into the medical profession helped, to a certain extent, to establish the fact that women's right to better health as well as to employment formed an essential component of the broader issue of social development. On the other hand, it must be remembered that these diverse forms of health care were available to a handful of fortunate women mostly residing in urban and semi-urban areas, while the majority of women were deprived of medical care by trained and qualified women doctors who were products of colonial medical education. The majority of Indian women suffered due to economic disadvantage. Medical care was economically out of reach for the poorer community. Widespread poverty, the lack of time to travel long distances to reach urban-based medical institutions, the fact that Western, Ayurvedic, and Unani medicines were more costly than folk forms of medicines, and the systematic discrimination against women in patriarchal society were a few of the hindrances that limited Indian women's access to and reliance upon formal medical aid.

APPENDIX 2A

Table 2A.1 List of Lady Students Who Passed Out of the CMC, Showing How They Were Employed

Names	Year (of passing)	Employment
Miss A. Niebel	1889	Under Dufferin Fund, Bhopal
Miss L.E. Sykes	1890	Unemployed, Calcutta
Miss T. Dissent	1890	Gone to England
Miss G.T. Pareira	1890	Dufferin Fund, Chittagong
Miss L.B. Smith	1890	Private practice, Calcutta
Miss J. Perry	1890	Dufferin Fund, Gaya
Miss L. Kirckpatrick	1890	Dufferin Fund, Hyderabad
Miss A. D'Souza	1890	Dufferin Fund, Amritsar
Miss Ida. M. Dissent	1890	Dufferin Fund, Allahabad
Miss W. Jahans	1890	Dufferin Fund, Cawnpore
Miss Ida Brown	1890	Dufferin Fund, Calcutta
Miss J.C. Muller	1891	Dufferin Fund, Delhi
Miss H. Forbes	1891	Dufferin Fund, Rangoon
Mrs M. Scott	1891	Dufferin Fund, Birhampore
Miss C. Brooking	1891	Dufferin Fund, Allighur
Mrs J.C. Smythie	1891	Dufferin Fund, Meerut
Miss L.M. Carroll	1893	Dufferin Fund, Agra
Miss E.L. Bridge	1893	Unemployed
Miss S.E. Bridge	1893	Unemployed
Miss M.S. Martin	1893	Calcutta Dufferin Hospital
Miss M.J. Watts	1893	Still studying at Medical College
Miss K. O'Byrne	1893	Nainital, Dufferin Hospital
Miss L.B. Long	1893	Bari Bouki under NWP, Dufferin Fund
Miss D.E. Pratt	1893	Dufferin Fund, Agra
Miss I. George	1893	Unemployed
Miss S. Anthony	1893	Unemployed
Miss A. Lisle	1893	Multan
Miss G. Woods	1893	Not known
Miss Mitter, M.B.	1890	Private practice, Calcutta
Miss B.M. Bose, M.B.	1890	Private practice, Calcutta
Miss B.B. Bose, M.B.	1891	Dufferin Fund, Cuttack

Source: From the principal, CMC, to the DPI, 30 March 1893, General Department, Education.

Table 2A.2 Female Pupils Who Graduated in 1890–1

Names	Employment
Sreemutty K.B. Guha	Private practice, Rungpur
Sreemutty Basanta Kumari Gupta	Private practice, Calcutta
Sreemutty Kiron Shoshi Mukerjee	Employed in Kumartuli Charitable Dispensary. Pay Rs 60. Rising to Rs 80. Free quarters + private practice allowed
Sreemutty Hemanginidebi	Bancoorah female hospital. Pay Rs 50. Free quarters + private practice allowed
Sreemutty Sarat Kumari Mitra	Private practice, Calcutta
Miss Shosji Mukhi (?)	Private practice, Dhaka
Miss Agnes Cecilia Basteen	Tipperah Zenana Hospital. Pay Rs 60. Free quarters + private practice allowed
Sreemutty Khiroda Sundari Roy	Dhankarbai Hospital, Nasik, Bombay. Pay Rs 100. Free quarters + private practice allowed
Mrs S.M. Biswas	Private practice, Calcutta

Source: From the principal, CMC, to the DPI, 30 March 1893, General Department, Education.

Table 2A.3 Female Pupils Who Graduated in 1891–2

Names	Employment
Sreemutty Harimati Dasi	Burdwan Female Hospital. Pay Rs 50. Free quarters + private practice allowed
Sreemutty Rajlakshmi Debi	Kandi Charitable Dispensary. Pay Rs 40. Free quarters + private practice allowed
Mrs Poospomoyee Sircar	Private practice, Calcutta

Source: From the principal, CMC, to the DPI, 30 March 1893, General Department, Education.

Table 2A.4 Female Pupils Who Graduated in 1892–3

Names	Employment
Sreemutty Priya Bala Guha	Employed under local board, Buckergubge
Mrs Kadambini Mukherjee	Sitapore Female Hospital, Oudh. Pay Rs 90. Free quarters + private practice allowed
Sreemutty Sushila Debi	Lady Dufferin Hospital, Bhagulpore. Pay Rs 60. Horse allowance Rs 15. Free quarters + private practice allowed
Sreemutty Bonotosini Chunder	Not known
Sreemutty Lokhi Moni Debi	Monghyrch Dispensary. Pay Rs 50. Free quarters + private practice allowed

Source: From the principal, CMC, to the DPI, 30 March 1893, General Department, Education.

Table 2A.5 Report of the Campbell Medical School for 1892–3

Sessions	Remained at the end of the sessions		Grand total	No. of students appearing at the final diploma exam		Percentage passed	
	M	F		M	F	M	F
1887–8	158		261	58		89.65	
1888–9	150	11	285	64		85.93	
1889–90	139	20	278	87		86.20	
1890–1	151	14	293	47	10	80.85	100
1891–2	136	17	293	43	4	97.67	75.00
1892–3	177	16	289	54	7	33.33	71.42

Source: By Brigade Surgeon Lieutenant Colonel S. Coull Mackenzie, MD, superintendent of the Campbell Medical School (in charge of the school throughout the year).

Notes and References

1. R.V. Parulekar, *Survey of Indigenous Education in the Province of Bombay, 1820–30* (Bombay: 1951); *Survey of Indigenous Education in the Madras Presidency, 1822–26*, reprinted in *The Beautiful Tree*, edited by Dharampal (New Delhi: Biblia Impex Pvt. Ltd, 1983). Cited in Aparna Basu, 'A Century

and a Half's Journey: Women's Education in India, 1850s to 2000', in *Women of India: Colonial and Post-Colonial Periods*, edited by Bharati Ray (New Delhi, Thousand Oaks, London: SAGE Publications, 2005), p. 184.

2. R.C. Mitra, 'Education', in *History of Bengal, 1757–1905*, edited by N.K. Sinha (Calcutta: University of Calcutta, 1967), p. 452.

3. Gail Minault, *Secluded Scholars: Women's Education and Muslim Social Reform in Colonial India* (New Delhi: Oxford University Press, 1998), p. 18.

4. Members of these new elite were in many cases descendants of the early indigenous collaborators of European merchant communities who ventured new opportunities and became opulent by serving the mushrooming European commercial houses in Calcutta as *banians* and diwans or business intermediaries. With the introduction of the permanent zamindari settlement, they became powerful proprietors of landed properties in Bengal, gaining further wealth and prominence.

5. Gyan Prakash, 'Science between the Lines', in *Subaltern Studies IX*, edited by Shahid Amin and Dipesh Chakrabarty (New Delhi: Oxford University Press, 1996). Quoted in David Arnold, *The New Cambridge History of India*, vol. 3, part 5, *Science, Technology and Medicine in Colonial India* (Cambridge: Cambridge University Press, 2000), p. 16.

6. Kapil Raj, 'Knowledge, Power and Modern Science: The Brahmins Strike Back', in *Science and Empire: Essays in Indian Context (1700–1947)*, edited by Deepak Kumar (New Delhi: Anamika Prakashan, 1991), p. 120.

7. Aparna Basu, 'The Indian Response to Scientific and Technical Education in the Colonial Era', in D. Kumar, *Science and Empire*, p. 126.

8. S.N. Sen, *Scientific and Technical Education in India 1781–1900* (New Delhi: Indian National Science Academy, 1991), p. 162.

9. According to historians, medical philanthropy and patronage in India sprang from a variety of motives. See David Arnold, *Colonizing the Body: State Medicine and Epidemic Disease in Nineteenth-Century India* (New Delhi: Oxford University Press, 1993), p. 269.

10. See Aparna Basu, 'Mary Ann Cooke to Mother Teresa: Christian Missionary Women and Indian Response', in *Women Missions: Past and Present*, edited by Fionna Bowie et al. (Oxford: Berg, 1993), p. 192. Cited in A. Basu, 'A Century and a Half's Journey', p. 185.

11. Meredith Borthwick, *The Changing Role of Women in Bengal, 1849–1905* (Princeton: Princeton University Press, 1984), p. 47.

12. Borthwick, *The Changing Role of Women in Bengal*, p. 49.

13. Some of the important historical works on Brahmo Samaj are as follows: Sivnath Sastri, *History of the Brahmo Samaj*, 2nd edition (Calcutta: Brahmo Mission Press, 1974); Meredith Borthwick, *Keshub Chunder Sen: A Search for*

Cultural Synthesis (Calcutta: Minerva Associates, 1977); and David Kopf, *The Brahmo Samaj and the Shaping of the Modern Indian Mind* (Princeton: Princeton University Press, 1979).

14. *Bamabodhini Patrika*, 6 April 1871, p. 92.

15. Borthwick, *The Changing Role of Women in Bengal*, p. 89. Mary Carpenter hoped that if educational opportunities were provided for young Indian girls and women, it might delay the age of marriage and, in the process, train 'native' females to be teachers, inspectors, and even medical doctors so that they might perform the work of 'uplift' for Indian and also British civilization themselves. See Antoinette Burton, 'From Child Bride to "Hindoo Lady": Rukhmabai and the Debate on Sexual Respectability in Imperial Britain', *The American Historical Review* 103, no. 4 (October 1998): 1119–46.

16. Geraldine Forbes, *The New Cambridge History of India*, vol. 4, part 2, *Women in Modern India* (Cambridge: Cambridge University Press, 1998), p. 43.

17. See Malavika Karlekar, 'Kadambini and the Bhadralok', *Economic and Political Weekly* 21, no. 19 (26 April 1986): WS-25–31.

18. Finance (Education), file no. 42, Proceeding 2–5, April 1875, pp. 103–5, West Bengal State Archives (WBSA).

19. Evidence of Koilash Chunder Bose, *Indian Mirror*, 13 August 1878. Cited in Borthwick, *The Changing Role of Women in Bengal*, pp. 321–2.

20. 'Female Doctors in Bengal', *Brahmo Public Opinion*, 27 June 1878.

21. Translated from Brajendranath Bandopadhyay's *Dwarakanath Gangopadhyay* (Calcutta: Bangiya Sahitya Parishad, 1952), p. 16. Cited in Malavika Karlekar, *Voices from Within: Early Personal Narratives of Bengali Women* (New Delhi: Oxford University Press, 1991), p. 170.

22. Mary Scharlieb, *Reminiscences* (London: Williams and Norgate, 1924), pp. 29–30.

23. Arnold, *Colonizing the Body*, p. 261.

24. Anil Kumar, *Medicine and the Raj: British Medical Policy in India, 1835–1911* (New Delhi: SAGE Publications, 1998), p. 59.

25. Proceedings of the Lieutenant Governor of Bengal, General Department, Education, July, 1883.

26. Proceedings of the Lieutenant Governor of Bengal, General Department, Education, July, 1883.

27. Letter from the DPI to the Principal, Medical College, Calcutta, proposing the admission of women, 5 May 1882, WBSA, General Education, March 1886, A 5–7. Cited in Samita Sen and Anirban Das, 'A History of the Calcutta Medical College and Hospital, 1835–1936', in *Science and Modern India: An Institutional History, c. 1784–1947*, edited by Uma Das Gupta, *Project of History of Science, Philosophy and Culture in Indian Civilization*, vol. 15, part 4 (2010), p. 498.

28. Letter no. 884 from A.W. Croft, Esq., DPI, to the secretary to Government of Bengal, 7 February 1884, WBSA, Education and Medical, June 1884, A 1–3, file 89-1.

29. 10 June 1882, WBSA, General Education, March 1886, A 5–7.

30. Proceedings of the Lieutenant Governor of Bengal, General Department, Education Branch, July 1883, 'Admission of Female Students into the Medical College', file 88-1/8.

31. Letter no. 472 from J.M. Coates, MD, Principal, Medical College to the DPI, 31 October 1882, WBSA, General Education, March 1886, A 5–7.

32. Proceedings of the Lieutenant Governor of Bengal, General Department, Education, March, 1886, file 31–8/9.

33. R. Harvey, WBSA, General Education, July 1883, A 9–10, file 88.

34. Note 84, A.P. MacDonnell, WBSA, General Education, July 1883, A 11, file 88.

35. Note 68, A.P. MacDonnell, WBSA, General Education, July 1883, A 11, file 88.

36. Proceedings of the Lieutenant Governor of Bengal, General Department, Education Branch, July 1883.

37. A.P. MacDonnell, WBSA, General Education, July 1883, A 11, file no. 88.

38. Proceedings of the Lieutenant Governor of Bengal, General Department, Education, March, 1886, file 31-8/9.

39. Letter no. 884 from A.W. Croft, Esq., Director of Public Instruction to the Secretary to Government of Bengal, 7 February 1884, WBSA, Education & Medical, June 1884, A 1–3, file 89-1.

40. Proceedings of the Lieutenant Governor of Bengal, General Department, Education, March,1886, file 31-8.

41. Proceedings of the Lieutenant Governor of Bengal, General Department, Education, April 1887.

42. Proceedings of the Lieutenant Governor of Bengal: File 21-6. Cited in *The Memoirs of Dr. Haimabati Sen: From Child Widow to Lady Doctor*, edited by Geraldine Forbes and Tapan Raychaudhuri (New Delhi: Roli Books, 2000), p. 23.

43. Proceedings of the Lieutenant-Governor of Bengal during November 1887, General Department.

44. Proceedings of the Lieutenant Governor of Bengal, General Department, Education, November 1887.

45. From Surgeon Major A. Crombie, Superintendent, Medical School, Dacca, to Secretary of Government of Bengal, July 1887, proceedings of the Lieutenant Governor of Bengal, General Department, Education.

46. Explicitly stated in Margaret I. Balfour, and Ruth Young, *The Work of Medical Women in India* (London: Oxford University Press, 1929).

47. Geraldine Forbes, *Women in Colonial India: Essays on Politics, Medicine, and Historiography* (New Delhi: Chronicle Books, 2005), p. 110.

48. *1901, Calcutta: Towns and Suburbs Census*. Cited in Borthwick, *The Changing Role of Women in Bengal*, p. 310n4.

49. H. Sharp, ed., *Progress of Education in India: 1907–1912, Sixth Quinquennial Review*, vol. 1 (Calcutta, 1914), pp. 151–2.

50. National Archives of India (NAI), Government of India, Home Department/Medical Branch, Deposit, July 1912.

51. Forbes and Raychaudhuri, *The Memoirs of Dr. Haimabati Sen*, p. 24.

52. Geraldine Forbes, 'Colonial Imperatives and Women's Emancipation: Western Medical Education for Indian Women in Nineteenth-Century Bengal', *Modern Historical Studies, Journal of the Department of History, Rabindra Bharati University* 2 (2001): 83–102; especially 94.

53. *Annual Report of the Medical Schools in Bengal 1914–1919* (Calcutta: Bengal Secretariat Press). Available at the National Library, Kolkata.

54. See Roger Jeffrey, *The Politics of Health in India* (Berkeley: University of California Press, 1988).

55. Cited in Geraldine Forbes, 'Medical Careers and Health Care for Indian Women: Patterns of Control', *Women's History Review* 3, no. 4 (1994): 519.

56. Forbes, 'Colonial Imperatives and Women's Emancipation': 91.

57. Report of the Bengal Branch of the Countess of Dufferin Fund for the Year Ending 30 November 1904 (Calcutta, Superintendent of Government printing), pp. 36–43. Available at National Library, Kolkata.

58. Forbes, *Women in Colonial India*, p. 112.

59. Geraldine Forbes, *Women in Modern India* (Cambridge: Cambridge University Press, 1996), p. 161. In the same year, that is, 1883, a Maharashtrian, Anandibai Joshee (1865–87) joined the Women's Medical College of Pennsylvania at Philadelphia in October 1883 and received her final degree in March 1886. She accepted the post of a lady doctor in the princely state of Kolhapur in the Bombay Presidency, but died before she could join (29 February 1887).

60. 'The Lady Dufferin Fund and the Indian Lady Doctor', *The Bengalee*, 7 February 1891, p. 65.

61. See Karlekar, 'Kadambini and the Bhadralok'; and also Karlekar, *Voices from Within*, p. 178.

62. Forbes and Raychaudhuri, *The Memoirs of Dr. Haimabati Sen*. Other writings on Haimabati include Forbes' *Women in Colonial India*; Indrani Sen, 'Resisting Patriarchy: Complexities and Conflicts in the Memoir of Haimabati Sen', *Economic and Political Weekly* 47, no. 12 (24 March 2012): 55–62;

Sujata Mukherjee, 'Women and Medicine in Colonial India: A Case Study of Three Women Doctors', *Indian History Congress Proceedings*, 66th Session, 2005–6, pp. 1184–91.

63. Borthwick, *The Changing Role of Women*, p. 325.

64. Borthwick, *The Changing Role of Women*, p. 325.

3 *Modernizing Reproductive Health*

Throughout the colonial period, traditional birthing practices and enlisting the assistance of birth attendants or dhais were attacked as unscientific by colonizers as well as elite Indians. Medical guidance was perceived as essential for improving and modernizing the physiological processes of maternity and childbirth. As pointed out in the last chapter, medical practitioners sometimes opposed the move to train women in Western medicine. Yet they almost always emphasized the urgent need to train and educate midwives in modern practices of birthing as well as prenatal and postnatal care.

Criticism of Indian birthing practices by the colonizers undoubtedly formed part of the 'otherization' of Indian cultural norms and bodily practices, and in upholding the superiority and scientificity of European practices. Modern reproduction was sought to be equated with science in general and biomedicine in particular. In this process of modernization of reproductive practices, the colonial authority, European and Indian practitioners of Western medicine, as well as social reformers were significantly involved. Colonial officials, medical professionals, missionaries, and private individuals focused particularly on the need to reform the practices of traditional birth attendants or dhais and to replace them by trained midwives. Many also perceived the urgency of creating new facilities for birthing women, including lying-in hospitals and modernizing the zenana by creating a new consciousness about pursuing hygienic practices during home birthing.[1]

Reforming the birthing process constituted a part of the corollary narratives of reformers' own attempts at self-modernization through embracing the trappings of science. Some groups, such as some nationalists, medical professionals, and some social reformers, embraced wholesale the science of colonialism and the West. There were other groups which wished to replace, and still others who desired to reinvigorate, Indian 'traditional' practices with scientifically informed tools. Many reformers sought to strike some sort of balance and advanced cautiously so that Western science, despite its spectacles of hygiene, did not get elevated to a degree that would smother India's cultural heritage or the vitality of its quotidian practices. It should also be stressed that dynamics of class and caste played a significant role in shaping the forces of modernization attempted through upgrading of birthing practices by introducing sanitary principles.

Medicalization of Childbirth

Quite early in the nineteenth century, an indigenous medical practitioner and teacher of medicine, Madhusudan Gupta, drew official attention to the necessity of reforming reproductive health by providing midwifery training to Indian women.[2] In his evidence before the Fever Hospital Committee (27 February, 4 March, 26 April, and 29 May 1837) he discussed—among other things—reproductive health in Bengal and pointed out that if a sufficient number of qualified female Hindu midwives were available at moderate charges, they would be able to accomplish a great deal by giving good advice to patients. He also pointed out that if a hospital with a lying-in ward was established where Hindu midwives and attendants could be employed then many married women of the interior castes would be able to attend that ward. This would save many lives. Moreover, he felt that if such a hospital could be united to a class in which an European professor of midwifery, well-acquainted with the vernacular language, would teach Hindu women that would bring in great benefit. Nothing came out of his proposal. However, the midwifery hospital of CMC, set up in 1840, gave training to male medical professionals in the use of modern techniques including forceps and ether to make deliveries easier.[3]

The number of female patients in the midwifery department showed an increase in the 1860s. Dr S.B. Patridge, the officiating principal of the CMC, wrote to Dr Hugh Macpherson, secretary to the principal inspector general, medical department: 'The Midwifery Department has made great progress; there have been no less than 131 confinements, much the largest number in any one year since the establishment of the institution.'[4]

Between 1875 and 1880, there was an increase of 27.29 per cent in the number of women patients of obstetric physicians at the CMC. The number of deliveries in various medical institutions in Calcutta including the Calcutta Medical College Hospital, General Hospital, Mayo Hospital and Dispensary, Campbell Hospital, Howrah General Hospital, and Municipal Police Hospital also rose from 247 in 1879 to 296 in 1880. Among the women in-patients in these hospitals, the number of native patients was the largest and among the native patients, East Indians formed the largest group. The number of women in-patients among the Europeans was the lowest. The lieutenant governor decided to establish a certain number of stipends to enable women to study midwifery in the wards. It was pointed out: 'There can be little doubt that the want of trained nurses in the interior of the country is severely felt.'[5] The number of in-patients treated by the obstetric physician at the CMC, however, showed a considerable decline in 1881, being only 1,008 against 1,277, 1,204, 1,238, 1,109, and 1,155 in the five preceding years.[6] At the Eden Hospital, which was devoted entirely to midwifery and diseases of women, the number of patients recorded an increase in 1887 than the previous year, but so did the number of deaths.[7] The number of deaths increased due to septicaemia in the hospital, as pointed out by Dr Harvey, the obstetric physician. He stated: 'There have been no less than 15 deaths from this cause alone—a cause which, according to modern theories, should never be found in a well-regulated hospital.'[8] However, in 1889 the total number of patients treated at the

Eden Hospital diminished owing entirely to the fact that the building was undergoing repairs for some months.[9]

Dhai: Colonial Critique and Ambivalence

In Bengal, as in other parts of India, childbirth was attended since precolonial days by indigenous midwives colloquially known as dhais. These traditional Indian midwives generally belonged to lower-caste Hindu or poor Muslim households, as higher-caste women would not incur the ritual pollution of childbirth.[10]

They were described as 'experienced and courageous women of advanced age and with clean clothes before whom she [the birthing mother] may not feel shy, who have cut their nails and who cheer her with friendly words.'[11] This view seems to be corroborated by the account of Lal Behari Day, who comments on the role of a village midwife who assisted in the birth of a child in the home of Badan, a peasant, thus:

> Rupá's mother—for she was the village midwife—was in all her glory. From the door of the lying-in room, into which no one, not even the father of the newly-born child, might enter—for it is regarded as ceremoniously unclean—she was every now and then showing the baby with evident pride and satisfaction, as if the newcomer were her own son or grandson.[12]

After the birth, the dhai played the important ritual role of cutting the umbilical cord with a sharpened piece of bamboo or shell covered with cow dung.[13] The duties of the dhai could extend from cutting the umbilical cord, washing the puerperal garments, and burying the placenta, to living in the home of the parturient mother and giving her and the infant regular massages and warm fomentations. Thus, they had to perform menial tasks but received meagre pay.

A familiar manoeuvre for imperial mentalities that increasingly envisaged India and all things Indian as essentially inferior and 'other' was traceable in identifying in 'Western' and 'Eastern' methods of childbirth one of the critical markers of difference between the East and the West. European doctors and missionaries believed that the dhai's methods were not only unclean and unscientific, but that she carried a heavy responsibility for the high rates of mortality in childbirth both among mothers and children. William Ward, a missionary from Serampore, drew attention to 'traditional customs of childbirth', which seemingly contributed to high maternal and infant mortality.[14] According to the description of a missionary author, in the practices of Bengali village midwives in the mid-nineteenth century, 'unscientific' and 'unchristian' customs seem to have been indistinguishable.[15]

The Madras Lying-in Hospital's prospectus in 1840 said: 'The great mortality of females in parturition from the barbarous treatment of Native practitioners is appalling [*sic*] to humanity, and calls forth the best feelings of those who have witnessed the sufferings of their fellow creatures, which might be obviated by the introduction of European treatment and practices.'[16]

Apart from the traditional birth attendants, another important target of attack was the unhygienic condition of the anturghar or sutikagriha where birthing took place. Generally, the smallest and darkest room in the house was the sutikagriha. Most European commentators, male or female, noted that childbirth was regarded both by Hindus and Muslims as ritually polluting, and, therefore, the lying-in chamber, or *chatthi ghar*, was a dirty shed or outhouse.

James Wise, the civil surgeon of Dhaka, in 1871, wrote a detailed account of the process of childbirth, which was associated with extreme pollution.[17] That was why the custom of seclusion within a lying-in room called the anturghar (often a makeshift hut of reed matting specially constructed for the purpose) was followed. A woman from one of the 'untouchable' castes was usually called in to cut the navel cord—a task so unclean that she would perform it with her left hand. This woman might attempt to speed labour in certain cases by such procedures as perineal massage. Women who had no professional attendants to help them in their labours were helped by relatives and neighbours.

Dr Stewart, a professor at the CMC, expressed his horror on seeing the 'filthy, smoky, and crowded hovels, to the straw of which the unfortunate Bengallee females are condemned by native usage in the hour of suffering'.[18] The situation did not change even after three decades. In 1876, the health officer for Calcutta gave a detailed account of traditional practices surrounding birthing:

> A chamber, a few feet square, so situated that at the best of times its atmosphere must be close, has every aperture carefully shut. It is crowded

> with relatives and attendants, so that there is often barely room to sit, and a fire of wood embers, or even charcoal, is burning in an open vessel. The atmosphere is principally smoke, which is increased by herbs scattered on the fire for the purpose. The woman is lying, generally on the ground, in the midst of this. The feeling on entering the room is that of impending suffocation.[19]

Margaret Balfour and Ruth Young, writing much later in 1929, pointed out that 'since bed and bedding are frequently burned after the event, the oldest of both are set aside for it'. Most nineteenth-century commentators merely noted the use of dirty rags without suggesting any reasons.[20]

In the first half of the twentieth century, continuation of the trend of tracing the causes of maternal and juvenile death and poor health to dirty midwifery and untrained midwives—apart from social customs, unhygienic environments, and malnutrition—was noticeably present in many accounts.[21] In 1901, the editors of the census commissioned a special inquiry into the methods of indigenous midwives. Some of the birthing practices followed in India and Europe were similar in many respects.[22] As many scholars have noted, over the course of the nineteenth century, earlier signs of European open-mindedness towards the peoples and cultures of India steadily faded and, in Metcalf's words, a 'stereotyped sense of Indian "difference"...loomed larger in the British imagination'.[23]

In an age when the process of othering became a governing principle in the shaping of colonial identities, ideologies, and practices, it was predictable that prevailing discourses denigrating the Indian practice of childbirth would follow the format of a 'dialogue with difference'.[24]

In the Census of India, 1911, the sutikagriha was described thus:

> The character of the room depends on the means and the enlightenment of the family, but generally it is one of the worst rooms in the house, or a shed is erected outside the compound. Among the poorer classes, the woman's accommodation is wretched. A portion of one of the living rooms may be screened off, or she may have to use the verandah; some doctors even state that the cowshed or the kitchen is occasionally used. As a rule, when a separate room is assigned, it is small, dark and ill-ventilated.[25]

To avoid evil spirits and also to protect the mother and child from catching a cold, windows and apertures were 'closed with mud or stuffed with old rags', which worsened the ventilation of the room.[26] Irrespective of the season, a small fire was kept burning in an earthen pot, which filled the room with smoke. During the first two decades of the twentieth century in Bengal, one in five babies died before their first birthday. In 1921, infant mortality rates were still on the increase. Among the bhadralok, it was double the corresponding proportions in England and other European countries.[27] During the decade ending 1885, the infant mortality rate in England was 142 per 1,000.[28]

It can be assumed from official records that maternal causes were responsible for over 60,000 female deaths in Bengal during 1921. Data obtained in a number of cases recently by the Department of Public Health suggest that ordinarily from 60,000 to 75,000 deaths among women were caused by prenatal, natal and postnatal conditions. A large number of women in these conditions fell victims to eclampsia, anaemia, and the postnatal conditions termed 'sutika'.[29] In 1931, 10,687 deaths from maternal causes were registered in Bengal, which rose to 11,525 deaths in 1932.[30]

It was reported in 1940 that infant mortality was higher in Bengal compared to any other province, except for the Central Provinces, Orissa, and Burma.[31] Among all the cities of the world, the infantile death rate was the highest in Calcutta.[32] The Calcutta Census of 1911 stated: 'The practice of cutting the umbilical cord with dirty instruments (e.g. a piece of split bamboo, or a conch shell) and of applying cow-dung ashes to the freshly cut end commonly results in tetanus neonatorum and causes a very large number of deaths among healthy infants every year.'[33]

Some European observers, particularly women doctors, praised the role of the dhai and expressed sympathetic views towards her, and even attributed her mishandling of delivery to ignorance rather than straightforward brutality. Christian missionaries like Elizabeth Beilby, for example, pointed out that Indian women were not entirely bereft of medical care. 'Their own women, dhais as they are called, can do something', she reported. She also pointed out that 'one or more of these women will always be sent for before an English lady doctor is called in'.[34] She mentions: 'I do not mean to say for a moment that all these women are essentially bad; but what I do maintain is, they are as ignorant of medical knowledge as a child who is just beginning to learn to read.'[35]

Even Dr Alice Marston, Beilby's successor at Lucknow, reported to an international missionary gathering: 'It is quite a mistake to suppose that Indian women are debarred from medical treatment altogether. From our point of view they are certainly debarred from sufficient or effectual medical aid; but from their own point of view they are, excepting in cases of special emergency, well provided for.'[36]

Mary Scharlieb once told Queen Victoria about 'the unintentional barbarities and injuries inflicted on these poor women by the kindly, but absolutely ignorant, native midwives.'[37] The feminist and educationalist Frances Hoggan described the dhai as a victim of Indian society thus: 'It is not to be wondered at that, low and degraded as is the position of Indian women at the present day, the untrained native Dhais or midwives should be ignorant, superstitious and incompetent in the extreme.'[38]

Due to the fact that it would be too expensive to replace the traditional birth attendant entirely by a new, trained class of modern, medicalized birth attendants, an ambivalence of colonial attitude towards them is also noticeable. Balfour and Young, practising medical women in India and authors of the most comprehensive account to date of women's medicine in India, described the dhai as 'the genius presiding over childbirth [whose] sway was undisputed', while at the same time criticized her for dangerous practices. Some doctors attempted to teach the dhai at least the rudiments of European training in midwifery and sanitation. Credit for the earliest attempts to train dhais is usually given to two classes that were opened in northern India, at Amritsar in 1866 and Bareilly the following year. The Amritsar school was founded specifically 'with the object of teaching native women—chiefly those of good caste.'[39] At the Bareilly school, at least until 1871, most pupils seem to have been unmarried orphans, many of them Indian Christians.[40] The Madras government embarked on a strategy of building up a body of Indian midwives trained in European methods. As pointed out by Sean Lang, this experiment can be accounted a success.[41] It was sustained, it maintained high medical standards, and it supplied a demand for trained midwives that was soon being expressed across India.

In Bengal, the Calcutta Medical College Hospital and the Mitford Hospital at Dhaka first opened courses for midwives in 1870.[42] Apparently, the midwifery training programme of the Eden Hospital (founded by the Lady Dufferin Fund) was better than that at many other provinces, since the Managing Committee of the North-Western Provinces' Branch of Lady Dufferin Fund sent there two female graduates of the Agra Medical School for the purpose of undergoing a more complete training in practical midwifery.[43]

The General Report of Public Instruction in Bengal reported that in the 1890s, the Eden Hospital trained an average of ten students a year. The midwifery course was apparently very tough and inconvenient to preclude traditional birth attendants from enrolling.[44] Since most of these programmes required knowledge of English and regular attendance, they did not attract traditional birth attendants.

The New Bhadralok and Birthing Reforms

Meredith Borthwick points out that from the middle of the nineteenth century the new bhadralok in Bengal showed eagerness to accept new knowledge of birthing, though it was accessible to those few who could afford its high cost.[45] In 1848, the report of the Midwifery Hospital announced that all of their six or more college graduates practising in Calcutta were 'habitually called to take charge of the women of the families they attend during their confinements, and that though not required to render manual assistance, except in cases of difficulty, they are always requested to undertake the medical management of every case, both during and after delivery'.[46]

Growth of lying-in facilities in different hospitals could in no way replace home birthing. It seems that the poor, low-caste women were sent to hospitals for childbirth, and many were sent by midwives only after complications had developed. Although the observation that the practice of confining women to filthy outhouses, filled with charcoal fumes, and heated by tisanes had been completely stopped by the native population of Calcutta was an over-optimistic remark, it may not be unreasonable to assume that many elite Indians were eager to accept new medical knowledge and professional help to facilitate home birthing.

The increasing influence of biomedical ideas was, no doubt, a corollary to the growth in the number of medical personnel whose arguments became more and more influential in dominating the ideas of childbirth. The steady expansion of a publishing industry in Calcutta and the suburbs facilitated the publication of numerous health manuals that found a ready market. Many of these writings were vernacular translations or adaptations of English-language guidebooks on birth management, childcare, and so on.[47] In 1857, an adaptation of Andrew Combe's *Treatise on the Physiological and Moral Management of Infancy* (1840) appeared under the title of *Sisupalan*, subtitled 'Infant Treatment', authored by Shib Chunder Deb.[48] The author suggested, among other things, that extensive changes should be made in arrangements for the sutikagriha. He recommended that it should be removed to a higher floor where conditions could be dry and sunny, facilitating ventilation of clean and fresh air.

Mohendracandra Gupta, in his book *Stribodh* (a manual of general instruction for women), stressed the importance of prenatal care.[49] Manuals on household hints and collections of essays for the purpose of female education sometimes contained sections on the health care for the child and mother.[50] In 1867, the *Bamabodhini Patrika* published a series of detailed and informative articles on midwifery, addressed to pregnancy, its symptoms and treatment, and delivery.[51] The first of a series of articles on midwifery in the *Bamabodhini Patrika* was on the sutikagriha, advising that it should be situated on the second storey of the house in a place that was neither too dark nor too windy. The room should have windows that allowed the passage of fresh air from north to south, should get plenty of sun, and be removed from any smelly, unsanitary places.[52] Many of the medical texts written for the use of students of the vernacular medical courses were widely read by the general public. These textbooks and manuals no doubt promoted the spread of biomedical ideas by presenting them in familiar and acceptable terms. A very notable and significant guidebook written in the Bengali language on midwifery, addressed to pregnant women themselves, was authored by a doctor, Jadunath Mukhopadhyaya, LMS of CMC in 1867 and was titled *Dhatrishiksha evam prasutishiksha arthat kathopakathan chhale dhai evam prasutidiger prati upadesh* (Guide to midwives and to mothers of newborn babies or advice to midwives and mothers of newborn babies through dialogue).[53] Jadunath noted that since so many women could read novels and plays, it was time for them to put their literacy to some practical use. The book, written in two volumes, went into seven editions. The seventh edition published in 1887 was a thoroughly enlarged and revised version of the old book. Jadunath dedicated the book to his teacher T. Edmondston Charles, Esquire, MD, professor of midwifery and diseases of women and children of CMC, 'as a token of gratitude and esteem for his high, professional acquirements'. About the background of this book, the author writes: 'My first child died because of the illiteracy and negligence of the dhai. I decided to write this kind of book so that no one from this country becomes the victim of such ill fate and suffers as a result from intolerable mental anguish.'

The author's stated aim was to teach 'practical midwifery' to illiterate midwives 'who are either quite ignorant of the art or have gained but a slightest experience in it, which can avail them nothing in the management of intricate cases'. Serious and fatal results often generally ensued from their ignorance. The author also maintained that the sheer existence of such a tract in the vernacular would motivate the illiterate midwives to try to read the book or get it read by someone else in order to master the practical lessons of their profession. For 'conveying knowledge to simple and unsophisticated minds', the author chose the style of the tract to be in the form of a dialogue. Jadunath was convinced that instead of a 'serious treatise' which could only be comprehended with the help of a teacher, his tract would be able to train the unsophisticated reader better, giving wider scope for entering into explanations.

The tract, which is divided into two parts, contains in the first part subjects like the duty of a midwife after entering the lying-in room, the management of the different stages of labour, the management of the parturient female, and proper nursing of the child till it is two years old. Many minute aspects of taking care of an infant were instructed on, including proper dressing, proper diet during the first three days including rules of breast feeding and timing of other nourishment, and rules of birthing. There was also advice on how far light as well as heat was necessary for the health and growth of the infant. It was emphasized that the baby had to be 'vaccinated within three months after birth'. The first part contained a chapter on 'Treatment of some of the most important diseases of children'. The second part of the book deals with subjects such as natural labour as well as abnormal cases with their treatments, puerperal haemorrhage, management of twin cases, signs of pregnancy, abortion and its consequent effects, and so forth. It is clear from this that the target readers were not illiterate native midwives only but also 'educated Hindu females'.

The book was admired and praised by doctors, the press, and some groups of Indians, including zamindars and even Bengali literary stalwarts like Bankim Chandra Chattopadhyay. The author recounts how when he mentioned his intention of writing this sort of a book to 'Babu' Saradaprasanna Mukhopadhyay, the zamindar of Gobordanga, he encouraged him and pointed out that this kind of book would benefit the country because many women who were educated at that time would become competent enough to be able to dispense the works of the dhai by reading his book. Dr Charles, Professor of midwifery and diseases of children at the Medical College, in a letter to the author dated 5 July 1870 (which was published in the 1887 edition of the tract), appreciated the merits of the book and observed (among other things):

> I am convinced that an extensive circulation of the book through the Bengalee districts in the Lower Provinces would do that amount of good which is possible, as long as the management of women in labour is entrusted to untrained women who can neither read nor write. I should much like to see every thana supplied with a copy as a commencement, and the inspection of police directed to encourage one or more dhayes to have the book read to them. Should it be found practicable to reach the women in this way, and it seems probable that the Dhayes would make an attempt to benefit by the means placed within their reach, such an experimental measure might be followed by a more extensive distribution of your work.

Opinions of the press were also very favourable. In the *Englishman* of 16 May 1870, it was pointed out that the medical graduates of the Calcutta University were a better educated lot than the old graduates of the Medical College and showed greater literary activity.

> To their industry and research is to be traced a promising medical literature in Bengali, which has sprang up within the last ten years. The work, which heads the present notice, is a very favourable specimen, written in an easy and colloquial Bengali, in the form of dialogues, intelligible to even a child of ten, it is calculated to prove not only an useful guide to Daees or midwives, but also a profitable companion to native mothers and nurses.... As the price of the book is only a rupee, there are few women of this class who cannot afford to purchase it. At the same time it would not be amiss if a copy were placed under the orders of the Government in each thannah, by which means it would be brought to the knowledge of those who never see even a vernacular newspaper.

It was also suggested that since the proper treatment of mothers and their children was a matter of national importance, the government might go a little out of its way to circulate the knowledge so conveniently arranged by Dr. Jadunath Mukherjee. The *Indian Daily News* reported (on 16 May 1870):

> It is satisfactory to notice that English education is in some respects being turned to account for the good of the people of this country. And we should like to see it bear more fruits used by Baboo Jadunath Mookherjee, Licentiate of Medicine and Surgery, Calcutta University, who has thrown into simple form, for popular use, the knowledge and esteem for that gentleman's professional acquirements. It must be gratifying to Dr. Charles to see that his instructions, in a matter of so much interest and importance to the uninformed women of India, have through one of his pupils, been made available for their advantage. The work is thrown into the form of simple dialogue in the vernacular, so that it may be read by almost all, or they may have it read to them. The work of Baboo Jadunath Mookherjee is on a subject affecting greatly the physical well-being of the people of India and there is no doubt it will be extensively useful.

Bankim Chandra Chattopadhyay, the well-known literati and editor of *Bangadarshan,* praised Jadunath for his *lokhitokorbrata* (dedication to people's welfare). He admired the method of writing as it could be comprehended by literate as well as illiterate women without help from an expert, and even pointed out that just as the *panjika* was thought to be indispensable for the Hindus as it helped them to find out about auspicious moments, this book was indispensable for life's well-being and should be acquired by every home.

Favourable opinions and admiration from a cross section of the society shows how medical personnel, colonial elite, and the educated Indian middle class were perceiving the importance of improving reproductive health practices by adopting new medical knowledge. It is also noteworthy that it was thought to be possible to educate and guide illiterate women belonging to lower classes and lower castes and engaged in practising midwifery, through vernacular texts without the help of an expert. But as time went on and other intricacies developed, this was thought to be an unattainable and inadvisable task.

At the beginning of the twentieth century, Sundarimohan Das (M.B., professor of midwifery at Physician and Surgeon College) wrote *Saral Dhatrisiksha* in B.S. 1308 (September 1901), in two parts. He was guided mainly by such standard works as Barnes' *Manual for Midwives* and Macnaughton-Jone's *Diseases of Women*. With regard to the subject of rearing of infants, Birch's *Management of Children* and *Food Disorders of Infants* were mostly followed. In the publisher's preface, it was written:

> A manual for midwives in simple and homely Bengali, wherein the subject matter is put so far as possible in relation to the ordinary experiences and practices of the people, is a long-felt want. An attempt in this direction was made 34 years ago [this was probably a reference to Jadunath's book] but since then, the science of obstetrics has made striking advances, discovering novel truths and discarding obsolete views.

It was mentioned that (Jadunath's) book no longer met all the requirements of the situation. *Saral Dhatrisiksha* was undertaken to remove this want, and since it combined an up to date knowledge of the literature on the subject with the author's extensive clinical experience ranging over two decades, it was expected that it would be found to be eminently serviceable to those for whom it was intended.

The subject matter was introduced in the form of dialogues and short stories. In several mofussil towns, medical men had to rely on the midwife, and the authors, therefore, attempted to acquaint her with the most common diseases of women. A few English terms were transliterated into Bengali and introduced in the dialogues with a view to help the midwives talk in intelligible ways with medical men. Particular care was taken to limit the province of the midwife while dealing with measures, and the clearest warning was in fact given against interfering in cases wherein qualified medical aid should be sought. The dangers of uncleanliness as leading to septic poisoning were very clearly pointed out, and repeated warnings were given against neglecting antisepsis, which would lead to the penalty of losing practice and license.

It was mentioned in the publisher's advertisement that part one aimed at educating housewives to enable them to deliver easily and to bring up the infant. Part two was intended for the dhais, to educate them about difficult labour and diseases of women. One notable feature, according to the publisher, was the repeated warnings issued to dhais by the author to not bring harm to the mother and the baby by committing the mistake of trying to handle complicated cases that were beyond their capacity. The author also very clearly outlined when it was imperative to consult a doctor. He even set certain norms of behaviour to be followed by the dhais in their interaction with the patients as well as the doctors. Another merit of the book, according to the publisher, was the simplicity of language which made it popular even among illiterate women. The use of occasional English words was not considered to be a negative feature since those words were commonly used, and if known, would help communication with doctors. Another positive attribute of the book, as stated, was that it was an outcome of the combination of authentic books on the subject and the author's experience of twenty years as a doctor.

Tracts on childcare and reproductive health written by medical personnel show how biomedicine was adapted to Indian practices. Besides following the imperative of reaching a wide section of Bengalis and influencing medical practices at homes through making it palatable/acceptable to a wide audience, the vernacular texts sought to incorporate certain traditional prejudices as well. The final result reflected a complex process of integration of the supposedly 'old' local epistemologies into an indigenized version of Western norms, an attitude that resonated with the reformers' aspiration to absorb selected elements of Western culture while conserving key elements of indigenous identity. The popularization and demand for hygienic home births heralded/reflected an articulation of medical modernity for India. As medical professionalism became more and more organized, the rhetoric of rationality increasingly became an important feature of the growing biomedical discourse.

Indian medical practitioners were sometimes engaged in adapting and modifying the received technical wisdom and practices of the West to suit particular needs of the Indian condition. This practice was not restricted to the arena of production of advice books. Modification of technical medical knowledge of the West to suit the specific needs of modernizing reproductive health in India was noticeable in the field of practical surgical obstetrics as well. Dr Kedarnath Das, the principal and professor of midwifery and gynaecology of Carmichael Medical College, prepared a *desi* version of the traditional Simpson forceps used in Great Britain for improved surgical intervention required in Indian birthing. He had observed that the pelvic area of the Bengali mother was generally seven-eighths of that of a British mother and the average weight of a Bengali baby was sixth-sevenths of that of a British baby. Based on this observation, he redesigned the traditional forceps to suit the requirements of Bengali mothers.[54]

The reform of reproductive health practices embraced changes not only in the field of medical ideas and practice, but also meant reorganizing the private space of the family as well. Familial structure was sought to be modified appropriately for modernizing reproduction. Within the traditional household structure, older women dominated reproduction-related customs and practices, which was no longer considered appropriate for facilitating modern reproductive practices. As pointed out by scholars, the wresting of the power to control reproductive matters from elder women was an aspect of transition 'that made the conjugal couple more central to the idealized "reformed" Bengali family'.[55] The presence of older women in the anturghar, who seemed to interfere with the process of birthing, was vehemently criticized by some because it became a hindrance in following practices based on scientific principles. In many vernacular texts, the dominance of the process of childbirth by older women was criticized and it was emphasized that control of childbirth was needed to be wrested out of the hands of these women.[56]

The reproductive reforms of the period were related to questions of caste identities and contributed to the formation of the middle-class identity in important ways. As pointed out earlier, the colonial state continuously harped on the 'dirty' and 'filthy' practices of the traditional birth attendants to assert its scientific superiority. Moreover, the dhais were accused of putting the mother's or infant's life in danger by interfering with the process of labour.[57] Upper-caste birthing customs were also subjected to vehement criticism, with a constant refrain of disapproval against the filthy environs in which birthing took place. Uncleanly 'native' habits were juxtaposed with Western hygienic practices and science-driven cleanliness. It would not be erroneous to argue that the concern of the new scientized bhadralok class for introducing reforms in birthing practices was one of the ways in which the upper caste/class shaped and articulated its identity as different from lower-caste/class people. Reforming birthing practices by attempting sanitization as part of medical professionalism meant that the control of birthing was sought to be wrested from lower-caste birth attendants, which helped in the formulation of middle-class identity by the appropriation of selected elements of Western knowledge.

For the upper castes in Bengal, as elsewhere, sanitized cleanliness became an ideology for asserting its own class identity as it worked in tandem with notions of caste purity and pollution.[58] In Bengal, the service of the traditional birth attendant belonging to the lower classes and castes was not entirely dispensed with, but only made much more marginalized. Emphasizing the concept of applying hygienic practices became very important for the self-definition of the middle class as well as for the otherization of the lower caste.

Though the upper-caste birthing room was depicted as unsanitary because of the superstitious ways of society, the dhai's association with dirt and the unclean quality of the old system of childbirth she represented was viewed as an aspect of her lower-caste status. The discourse on cleanliness, in the hands of reforming Bengali men, became a tool to limit the role of the dhai and locate her firmly in her low place, and represented an ambition of asserting an upper-caste identity differentiated from the lower castes, yet which was hegemonic over them. Thus, the language of sanitation was used to work out the class and caste differentiation between layers of indigenous society itself. The upper class' attempts at modernizing reproductive practices involved the reordering of social hierarchy in a way that would wrest control over women's bodies from the low-caste poor dhais and open up new professional spaces.

The midwifery training programmes in different teaching hospitals attracted *bhadramahilas* (gentlewomen), and midwifery became a feasible career for many of them. The opinion voiced by Keshab Chandra Sen in 1883 found many supporters:

> To us Indians, in the present state of Native Society, lady MD's are an expensive luxury which may possibly be excluded from all serious consideration at least for some time to come, but competent midwives are to us a necessity which cannot be dispensed with. Indian women do not die because of the absence of female doctors possessed of high University honors, but deaths, miserable and horrible, have actually resulted from the want of good midwives. It is this great question, therefore, which,

> affecting, as it does, the lives of thousands of the Native population, must be faced and solved by all reformers and philanthropists as the most pressing question of the day in India.[59]

Despite some initial apprehensions, many Brahmo and Hindu women showed eagerness to enrol for the midwifery training course of the CMC and embraced the profession quite happily. In 1879, Srimati J.L. Ghosh and Srimati T.M. Ray, 'midwives, holding diploma of the Calcutta Medical College Hospital', advertised their practice at 103 College Street, Calcutta, in the pages of *Brahmo Public Opinion*.[60] By 1880, there were about half a dozen trained midwives practising in Calcutta. Their success attracted others from the mofussil.

In 1898, the Tippera District Board, very dissatisfied with its European lady doctor, felt that it would be more beneficial to the local community to have a skilled midwife. In the same year, the Board considered opening a midwifery class, to be taught by the lady doctor of the zenana hospital in Comilla as her hospital workload was not very heavy. The District Board of Contai was advised to appoint a midwife who could also serve as teacher of the local girls' school to save extra expenses.[61]

Some of the members of the Saroj Nalini Dutt Memorial Association (SNDMA) at the district and village levels excelled at midwifery. Nalinibala Devi, whose father and husband were both doctors, learnt midwifery from her family. In Sylhet, she founded a Mahila Samiti and a clinic and herself arranged forceps deliveries.[62] Hemangini Sen, founder member of the Tala Mahila Samiti, herself taught and practised midwifery.[63] Some like Charusila Devi, secretary of the Jaduboyra Samiti, came from an orthodox family but acted as midwife to low-caste women and also provided a well-ventilated room in her own house to be used as an anturghar by poor local women.[64]

***

The regime of cleanliness that accompanied science allowed the members of the elite class to transmute dirt, filth, and pollution as qualities associated with the lower castes, viewed as the 'others'. The need to control the fertility and reproductive capacity of middle-class women, and separate them from those designated low and dangerous, thus, opened the doors for some upper-caste women to undertake what was hitherto seen to be the polluting work of bringing children into the world. Breaking the taboo of pollution associated with childbirth was accompanied by the process of making uncleanliness a quality intrinsic to some 'other' members of society. Women of higher castes thus gained new careers and public spaces, while also losing, to some extent, older relationships spread across caste and religious boundaries.

In urban areas like Calcutta, women seeking medical help in birthing often seemed to prefer attending the zenana hospitals and maternity homes run by the Corporation of Calcutta than the more prestigious Eden and Carmichael Hospitals. The Calcutta Corporation's scheme of providing trained domiciliary midwives, backed by a chain of subsidized maternity homes introduced in 1916, became successful to a certain extent. In 1922, the Corporation staff handled 3,917 maternity cases (more than a fifth of the babies born in Calcutta). There were only five maternal deaths. The Health Officer of Calcutta claimed that this was a remarkable achievement for four women health visitors and sixteen midwives, 'specially in view of the fact that most of the cases were delivered on "kutcha" floors of bustee huts under the most appalling sanitary conditions'.[65] The prestigious hospitals suffered the disadvantage of being teaching institutions, where medical students attended or witnessed most of the cases—a practice to which many of the patients objected.[66] Institutionalized reproductive health became a major site of medical contest between the colonial power and Indian medical profession. Indian training in obstetrics and gynaecology was severely criticized, subsequently leading to the withdrawal of recognition by the General Medical Council in 1921. This was interpreted by Indian medical men as an instance of racial prejudice.[67] Indian medical men, including Kedarnath Das and Nilratan Sircar, challenged the official statistics.[68] Indians also argued that if available cases were better utilized, the problem of 'defective midwifery' could easily be resolved. Sir Patrick Hehir, the director-general of medical services, seemed to concur when he referred to reports that Indian midwives in the hospitals sympathized with their patients. Students allotted to particular cases were often not sent for by the midwife concerned.[69]

In the increasingly politicized atmosphere of the 1920s and the 1930s, modern midwidfery was linked to the progress of the Indian community and became a matter of national pride.[70] Various reports of the 1920s, particularly the report of the health officer in the municipal administration of Calcutta of 1922, discuss the impact of seclusion, which was now seen as a solely Muslim practice relating to the reproductive and general health of women. The Bhore Committee Report of 1946 carried a note of dissent by three Muslim doctors who questioned the attribution of ill health in general, and of tuberculosis in particular, to the practice of purdah.[71] Thus, reproduction was constituted and reconstituted not only in the medical arena but in political and social reform agendas over the course of the second half of the nineteenth and the first half of the twentieth centuries. It did stand in for larger entities and formed a part of colonial administrative or medical practice, and was simultaneously a constituent in the representational politics of nation, community, caste, and family.

As pointed out by Sara Hodges, the invocation of reproduction as an object of reform relies on the productive slippage between society and biology. This slippage actually enabled reproduction to be a potent site for reformist efforts. Reproduction as an issue was closely bound up with the self-perceptions and the need for desired self-perpetuation of the new middle classes of Bengal. Women as reproducers and mothers were required to provide for a progeny masculine and muscular enough to combat colonialism, fulfil the ambitions of nationalism, and fill the need for greater numbers of strong and forceful religious communities.

In the early part of the twentieth century, the issue of national efficiency became part of the constitutive element in the attempted reform of reproductive health. Debates about maternal and child health were linked to concerns regarding not only diseases and death, but also to questions of family planning, to address the problem of so-called overpopulation and increasing national efficiency, which became part of the political agenda of women's organizations as well. This discussion forms the subject matter of another chapter.[72]

Notes and References

1. Some of the important works on reproductive health in colonial India are as follows: Dagmar Engels, *Beyond Purdah? Women in Bengal 1890–1939*

(New Delhi: Oxford University Press, 1996); Geraldine Forbes, 'Managing Midwifery in India', in *Women in Colonial India: Essays on Politics, Medicine, and Historiography*, by Geraldine Forbes (New Delhi: Chronicle Books, 2005), pp. 79–100; Sean Lang, 'Drop the Demon Dai: Maternal Mortality and the State in Colonial Madras, 1840–1875', *Social History of Medicine* 18, no. 3 (2005): 357–78; Sara Hodges, ed., *Reproductive Health in India: History, Politics, Controversies* (New Delhi: Orient Longman, 2006); Charu Gupta, *Sexuality, Obscenity, Community: Women, Muslims and the Hindu Public in Colonial India*, second impression (New Delhi: Permanent Black, 2008); Arabindo Samanta, 'Physicians, Forceps and Childbirth: Technological Intervention in Reproductive Health in Colonial Bengal', in *Medicine and Colonialism: Historical Perspectives in India and South Africa*, edited by Poonam Bala (London: Pickering & Chatto, 2014), pp. 111–26.

2. He was born in a Vaidya family of Baidyabati in Hooghly district. In 1826, he entered the newly started Ayurvedic medicine classes at Sanskrit College, and in 1835, he entered the CMC. He is credited as being among the first ones to overcome caste prejudices and perform dissection on the human body.

3. See Chapter 1.

4. Proceedings of the Lieutenant Governor of Bengal, General (Medical) Department, April 1862.

5. Proceedings of the Lieutenant Governor of Bengal during June 1881, Medical and Municipal Department, Calcutta, 1881.

6. Proceedings of the Lieutenant Governor of Bengal, June 1882, Medical and Municipal Department, June 1882.

7. 1,607 patients were treated during 1887 against 1,541 in the previous year. Of these, 946 were Europeans, including 33 remaining on 1 January, among whom there were 39 deaths. In 1886, 957 were treated, with 28 deaths. In 1886 and 1887, 584 and 661 natives respectively were treated. The daily average of both classes was 67.8, against 74.1 in 1886. The number of deaths increased to 58 against 40. See *Report of the Calcutta Medical Institutions for the year 1888*, available at the National Library, Kolkata.

8. *Report of the Calcutta Medical Institutions for the year 1888.*

9. *Report of the Calcutta Medical Institutions for the year 1889.*

10. In Bengal, she could be a member of the hadi or dom castes; in north India she was generally a chamar or of the sweeper caste. In the south, she was of the barber caste. See S.C. Bose, *The Hindoos as They Are: A Description of the Manners, Customs and Inner Life of Hindoo Society in Bengal* (Calcutta: W. Newman, 1881), p. 23; Meredith Borthwick, *The Changing Role of Women in Bengal, 1849–1905* (Princeton: Princeton University Press, 1984), p. 155; C. Gupta, *Sexuality, Obscenity, Community*, p. 177.

11. Dr Julius Jolly, *Indian Medicine*, trans. from German by C.G. Kashikar (New Delhi: Munshiram Manoharlal, 1994[1951]), p. 69.

12. Lal Behari Day, *Bengal Peasant Life* (Calcutta: Editions Indian, 1970 [1874]), p. 21. Also cited in Forbes, *Women in Colonial India*, p. 83n19.

13. Dagmar Engels, 'The Politics of Childbirth: British and Bengali Women in Contest, 1890–1930', in *Society and Ideology: Essays in South Asian History*, edited by Peter Robb. (New Delhi; Oxford University Press, 1993), pp. 222–46.

14. See, for example, William Ward, *A View of the History, Literature and Mythology of the Hindoos Including a Minute Description of their Manners and Customs* (Serampore: Mission Press, 1818), pp. 115–16. Also cited in Supriya Guha, 'The Best Swadeshi": Reproductive Health in Bengal, 1840–1940', in Hodges, *Reproductive Health in India*, p. 140.

15. Editors' introduction to excerpts from Hannah Catherine Mullens, 'Phulmani o Karunar Bibaran', in *Women Writing in India, vol. 1: 600 BC to the Present*, edited by Susie Tharu and K. Lalitha (New York: Feminist Press, 1991), p. 205.

16. Oriental and India Office Collection (OIOC), P/247/53 Madras Pub. Proc., 8 August 1840. In 1829, the *Lancet* deplored high maternal and infant death rates as results of the 'violent measures in use by these uninstructed persons [dais]'. See *Lancet* (1829) ii, p. 760. Also cited by Lang, 'Drop the Demon Dai': 365.

17. See Guha, 'The Best Swadeshi', pp. 41–2. Government of Bengal, *Report on the Charitable Dispensaries*, 1871, File V/24, India Office Collection, British Library. Also, unpublished monograph by James Wise, *Notes on the Races, Castes and Tribes of Eastern Bengal*, pp. 50–2, 142.

18. Dr Stewart, *Report on the Statistical History of the Female Hospital*, GRPI for 1846–7, Appendix E, no.10, p. clxxv. Also cited in Borthwick, *The Changing Role of Women in Bengal*, p. 154.

19. Bengal Census 1881, part II, p. 120. Also cited in Borthwick, *The Changing Role of Women in Bengal*, p. 154.

20. Margaret I. Balfour and Ruth Young, *The Work of Medical Women in India* (London: Oxford University Press, 1929), pp. 126–7.

21. Balfour, *The Indian Year Book, 1922*, p. 483. Cited in Kabita Ray, *History of Public Health: Colonial Bengal 1921–1947* (Calcutta: K.P. Bagchi & Company, 1998).

22. See Engels, *Beyond Purdah? Women in Bengal*, p. 129.

23. Thomas R. Metcalf, *Ideologies of the Raj* (Cambridge: Cambridge University Press, 1994), p. 24.

24. The phrase 'dialogue with difference' comes from Elizabeth M. Collingham, *Imperial Bodies* (Cambridge: Polity Press, 2001), p. 6.

25. Cited in Engels, *Beyond Purdah? Women in Bengal*, p. 125.

26. Cited in Engels, *Beyond Purdah? Women in Bengal*, p. 125.

27. *Census of India, 1921*, vol. 1, pp. 209, 230. Cited in Engels, *Beyond Purdah? Women in Bengal*, p. 128.

28. *Census of India, 1921*, vol. 1, p. 209. Cited in Engels, *Beyond Purdah? Women in Bengal*, p. 128. The rate improved rapidly after 1900 and in 1920 became as low as 80 per 1,000.

29. *54th Annual Report of the Director of Public Health for Bengal: 1921*. It was commented in the above report that pregnancy or childbirth directly or indirectly influenced deaths among females during the childbearing period to the extent of 8 to 10 per cent of those under 15 years of age, 50 to 60 per cent of those between 15 to 20 years, 30 to 33 per cent of those between 20 to 30 years, and 3 to 4 per cent of those above 40 years of age.

30. *Bengal Public Health Report for the Year 1932*, by Dr R.B. Khambata, Department of Public Health, Government of Bengal.

31. Resolution no. 1176 Public Health., dated 23 July 1940, of the Government of Bengal, Department of Public Health and Local Self-Government.

32. *54th Annual report of the Director of Public Health for Bengal: 1921*.

33. *Census of India*, 1911, vol. 6, part 1, p. 30, cited in Dagmar, *Beyond Purdah? Women in Bengal*, p. 129.

34. John Lowe, *Medical Missions: Their Place and Power* (Edinburgh: Oliphant, Anderson and Ferrier, 1886), p. 191. Quoted in Rosemary Fitzgerald, '"Making and Moulding the Nursing of the Indian Empire": Recasting Nurses in Colonial India', in *Rhetoric and Reality: Gender and the Colonial Experience in South Asia*, edited by Avril A. Powell and Siobhan Lambert-Hurley (New Delhi: Oxford University Press, 2006), p. 198.

35. E. Beilby, 'Medical Women for India', *Journal of the National Indian Association* 176 (August 1885): 357–65, 358.

36. Alice K. Marston, 'Medical Work for Women in the Mission-field', in *Report of the Centenary Conference on the Protestant Missions of the World*, vol. 2, *9–19 June 1888*, edited by J. Johnson (London: James Nisbet and Co., 1888), p. 147. Cited in Fitzgerald, 'Recasting Nurses in Colonial India', p. 199.

37. M. Scharlieb, *Reminiscences* (London: Williams and Norgate, 1924), p. 91.

38. *Englishwoman's Review* 144 (April 1885), p. 150. However, the journalist Mary Billington, writing in 1895, mentioned 'ignorance, cruelty, and avarice' as the characteristics of dhais. M.F. Billington, *Women in India* (London: Chapman and Hall, 1895), p. 3.

39. OIOC P/273, *Madras Public Proceedings*, 26 March 1872, no. 103. Also cited in Lang, 'Drop the Demon Dai'.

40. OIOC P/276, *Madras Public Proceedings*, 26 May 1875, no. 95; *Lancet* (1874) i, p. 287.

41. OIOC P/276, *Madras Public Proceedings*, 26 May 1875, no. 95; *Lancet* (1874) i, p. 287.

42. 'Dhatri bidyalayer bibaran', *Bamabodhini Patrika* 6, no. 89 (January 1871). Also cited in Borthwick, *The Changing Role of Women in Bengal*, p. 159.

43. *Report of the Calcutta Medical Institutions for the year* 1887, 18 July 1888, Calcutta.

44. Geraldine Forbes points out: First, midwifery candidates had to complete 'the Sick Nursing Certificate' programme. This programme was open to women of over seventeen, with a vernacular or Anglo-vernacular Lower Primary certificate, a certificate of good moral character, and a probationary residency of six months. The examination for this certificate tested knowledge and practice of elementary sanitation; bed-making; use of local remedies such as poultices, cold-water dressing, and so on; various kinds of baths; application of bandages, slings, and splints; administration of medicines; observation of conspicuous symptoms; and diet preparation. Candidates were required to take a course in anatomy (female pelvis and the organs, and other structures concerned in parturition), signs and symptoms of pregnancy and natural labour, indications of simple and complex labour, treatment of excessive haemorrhage, breastfeeding, and management of the newborn infant. In addition to theoretical and practical exams, each candidate was required to assist a doctor at twenty confinements and deliver three infants independently. See *The Countess of Dufferin's Fund—the Sixth Annual Report of the National Association for Supplying Female Medical Aid to the Women of India, Burma Branch, for the Year 1892* (Calcutta: Office of the Superintendent of Government Printing, 1893), pp. 13–14. Also cited in Geraldine Forbes, 'Colonial Imperatives and Women's Emancipation: Western Medical Education for Indian Women in Nineteenth Century Bengal', *Modern Historical Studies* 2 (March 2001): 83–102, 86.

45. Borthwick, *The Changing Role of Women in Bengal*, pp. 156–7.

46. *General Report on Public Instruction* for 1847–8, Appendix E, no. VII, p. cl. Also cited in Borthwick, *The Changing Role of Women in Bengal*, p. 157n24.

47. For an excellent analysis of the world of daktari prints, see Projit Bihari Mukharji, *Nationalizing the Body: The Medical Market, Print and Daktari Medicine* (London, New York: Anthem Press, 2009), pp. 75–110.

48. Shib Chunder Deb, *Sisupalan*, part 1 (Serampore: 1857); part 2 (Calcutta: 1862). Also see Chapter 4 of this volume.

49. Mohendracandra Gupta, *Stribodh* (Dhaka: 1862). Also cited in Borthwick, *The Changing Role of Women in Bengal*, p. 161.

50. For a detailed discussion, see Chapter 4 of this volume.

51. *Bamabodhini Patrika* nos 3 and 4 (1867–8): 8 (1872).

52. 'Dhatribidya', *Bamabodhini Patrika* 3, no. 52 (December 1867). Also cited in Borthwick, *The Changing Role of Women in Bengal*, p. 161.

53. Jadunath Mukhopadhyaya, *Dhatrishiksha evam prasutishiksha arthat kathopakathanchhale dhai evam prasutidiger prati upadesh* (Chinsura: Chikitsabodhak Press, 1875 [1867]).

54. See Samanta, 'Physicians, Forceps and Childbirth'.

55. Also see Chapter 4 of this volume.

56. See Gangaprasad Mukhopadhyaya, *Matrishiksha* (Calcutta: United Press, 1902); Haridhan Datta, *Narijibane dehatattva o svasthya vishayak sadharaner pathyopayogi pustak* (Calcutta: Chakrabarti & Co., 1906).

57. *Native Female Medical Education in Bengal, the N.W. Provinces and Oudh and the Punjab*, Home-Medical, 76/83, December 1887, National Archives of India, New Delhi. Cited in Anshu Malhotra, 'Of Dais and Midwives: "Middle Class" Interventions in the Management of Women's Reproductive Health in Colonial Punjab', in Hodges, *Reproductive Health in India*, pp. 199–226, 208.

58. Anshu Malhotra finds that the introduction of new, or seemingly new, midwifery practices appealed to the emerging middle-class elites of colonial Punjab, in part to replicate the colonial state's attack on 'native' or 'low-caste' dhais as backward, dangerous, and menacing. The attack on dhais, as articulated by the Punjabi middle classes, was an aspect of the way in which the new middle classes, as upper-caste elites, were defining themselves and shaping their identity. One of the elements of the middle-class identity among different communities (the Hindus and the Sikhs) was their upper-caste status. At a very basic level, then, control over fertility meant sequestering women from the reach of the lower-caste dhais at the time of childbirth. Not only did the Punjabi elite begin to share with the colonial state notions of hygiene, cleanliness, and the propagation of science, but also transformed these to the disadvantage of those who provided them with customary services, including the dhai.

59. Letter from Keshab Chandra Sen, *New Dispensation*, 9 December 1883. Cited in Borthwick, *The Changing Role of Women in Bengal*, p. 327.

60. Borthwick, *The Changing Role of Women in Bengal*, p. 327.

61. Borthwick, *The Changing Role of Women in Bengal*, p. 328.

62. 'Nalinibala Devi', *Banga Laksmi*, 1334–5, pp. 691–2. Also cited in Engels, *Beyond Purdah? Women in Bengal*, p. 149.

63. 'Hemangini Sen', *Banga Laksmi*, 1334–5, pp. 615–18.

64. *Saroj Nalini Dutta Memorial Association* (SNDMA) *Report*, 1927, p. 50. Also cited in Engels, *Beyond Purdah? Women in Bengal*, p. 149.

65. *Report of the Health Officer in the Municipal Administration of Calcutta, Corporation of Calcutta.*

66. See comments by Rai Bahadur Dr Chunilal Bose and response by Dr Alice Headwards in 'Discussion on Organisation of Child Welfare Work', *Proceedings of the Seventh Congress of the Far Eastern Association for Tropical Medicine, Calcutta, December 1927* (Calcutta: Government of India Press, 1928), pp. 847, 857.

67. This was the view expressed by Dr B.C. Roy, then professor of medicine at the Carmichael Medical College, Calcutta, in his presidential address to the All India Medical Conference at Lahore in December 1929.

68. See Anonymous, 'The Problem of Midwifery Training in Indian Medical Colleges', *The Calcutta Medical Journal* 19, no. 3 (1924): 158–60; and 'Presidential Address of Dr. B.C. Roy, All India Medical Conference, Lahore, December 1929', *Journal of the Indian Medical Association* 1, no. 1 (March 1930): 3–4.

69. 'Presidential Address of Dr. B.C. Roy', p. 26.

70. 'Few people would dispute that midwifery was the keystone in a nation's progress.' 'Presidential Address by Dr. A.L. Mudaliar', in *Proceedings of All India Medical Conference*, Delhi, 1934. Also see S. Guha, 'The Best Swadeshi'.

71. See note by A.H. Butt, Khadija Shuffi Tyabji, and M.A. Hameed in the *Report of the Health Survey and Development Committee under the Chairmanship of Sir Joseph Bhore* (Delhi: Government of India Press, 1946), vol. 1, p. 18.

72. See Chapter 5 of this volume.

4 *Sexuality, Domesticity, and Health Advice for Women*

Throughout the nineteenth century, colonial urban centres of India such as Calcutta witnessed the publication of numerous vernacular texts, including domestic manuals, guide books, pedagogical writings, and essays in different periodicals, on a variety of subjects. This corpus of writing included a large number of publications on the subject of health and diseases and many of these writings separately included discussions on—among other topics—the physical condition of Bengalis. They reflected the middle-class Hindu Bengali's concern and anxiety about the supposed continuous deterioration of health of the nation in general and of the Bengali community in particular.

In many writings, the starting point of the discussion on national health was the physical weakness and lack of strength of Indians, especially Bengalis, even though there was a complementary view that the Bengali was second to none in intelligence. The causes of this supposed deterioration of health of the Bengalis and the measures to be adopted to improve health conditions were the subject matter of intense debate and discussion in a number of essays.[1] There emerged a socio-medical rhetoric of degeneration, emphasizing that the question of how best to preserve or restore health should be regarded as a matter of urgent national security, requiring immediate attention.

One author pointed out in an essay titled 'The Revival of National Health', published in a periodical called *Chikitsa Sammilani*: 'Most foreigners and some thinking Indians strongly believe that the people of our country have a frail body and a short lifespan, and that is certainly not far from truth.'[2] It was further stated that despite being equal in mind, Europeans are superior to Bengalis in terms of physical constitution and strength. In their attempts to find reasons for this, many writers opined that adoption of wrong habits, including Western food and drinking habits, had an adverse impact on health.

According to some observers, the reasons behind such declining status of health could be grouped under two broad heads, namely: (*a*) natural or local and (*b*) gradual pollution induced.[3] It was also argued that natural or local factors like environment, climate, and so forth were hard to be eliminated. Many middle-class Bengalis of the time, in fact, were influenced by an environmental determinism promoted by the miasmatic theories and the medico–topographical surveys carried out by Europeans since the early nineteenth century.[4] Different medical investigations of climate and topography contributed towards fashioning the idea of a pathogenic Bengal. Bengal's uncongenial environments seemed to encourage diseases like malaria. It was described as an 'emasculating disease' that threatened reproduction, rendered individuals weak and sickly, and thus seemed to accentuate the division (already entrenched in colonial ideology and practice) between the 'manly' and 'martial' races of the north and northwest and the 'effeminate' Bengalis.

The census reports of 1891 and 1901 fuelled the perception that middle-class Bengali Hindus were a 'dying race' being decimated by malaria, while the Muslims of eastern Bengal, where malaria was less prevalent, continued to multiply.

Health, Marriage, and Sexuality

No less harmful for health were some of the prevailing social customs as well as harmful habits. The hope was expressed that changes which resulted from pollution or harmful practices and made the physique weak and fragile could be controlled through individual will or reform of damaging social norms. Some major factors identified as harmful for health were listed as '(*a*) child marriage, (*b*) multiple marriage, (*c*) improper food habits, (*d*) lack of physical exercise, (*e*) alcoholism, (*f*) masturbation and nocturnal pollution, and (*g*) indiscriminate coital indulgence'.[5]

One major cause of concern was the ill effects of child marriage on the health of young husbands and wives, as well as their offspring. It was stated:

> Some Hindus and many Muslims of this country get married at a very young age. Among the Hindus, girls eight/nine years old get married to boys 11/12 years old. Marriage at such a young and immature age results in the girls having their first issues around the age of 11/12; being as feeble and fragile as their parents, these babies either do not live long, or grow up to be weak and sickly. Second, the girl-mothers face a lot of problems during pregnancy and difficulties and pain at the time of delivery often leading to maternal mortality. Third, even if these girls are spared their lives during childbirth, they become subject to a lifetime of ill health.[6]

At the beginning of the twentieth century too a great deal of emphasis was put on the intimate relation between marriage and health. It was pointed out in an essay published in *Swasthya*: 'When entering into matrimony one must always remember one's responsibilities for the nation's health and the fact that health and marriage are inextricably linked.'[7] It was also stated that:

> It was usually seen that children of healthy parents are strong and healthy, whereas weak children result from a marriage between parents in poor health. National health depends upon the national system of marriage, and this will always be the case. An example of this relationship is the present state of the English, French or other European nationalities—if we compare the state of our health with theirs, it will be easy to understand how depressed our state is compared to theirs. There is not a whit

> of doubt that the difference in our health and theirs is the result of the system of marriage.[8]

With the progress of the discussion on medical science, discussions on sexuality (which involved focusing on the relation between different sexual practices and health) also began to appear frequently in vernacular writings. The concept of sexuality—as it developed in the nineteenth century—was closely related to the declared goal of heterosexual relations on the one hand and national health on the other. Different writings advocated that production of children was the sole aim of the sexual union of husband and wife and that uncontrolled sexual union between husband and wife might lead to decline of health. The writer of *Baigyanik Dampatya Pranali* stated:

> The sexual union which produces children is described as the true satiation of sensual proclivities. The satiation of the senses affects every part of the body, physical and mental well-being are greatly decreased, and as a result the basic material of which the body is composed is lost and destroyed. The satiation of the senses is in itself harmful, whether in excess or in a balanced manner, whether at the proper or the improper time, whether out of necessity or out of desire, the satiation of the senses will definitely lead to a loss of physical health.[9]

Controlled sexual intercourse between men and women was proclaimed as the divine rule. It was argued:

> Since the organs meant for procreation do not help the body in any way, the functions related to those organs, including coitus between men and women, also do not help the body in any way; but if such activities including coitus cross the sanctified limits and become perverted, then they harm the body, and that is why it is necessary to abide by God's rules.[10]

Sometimes opinions of European doctors were also cited in this and other matters relating to sexual practices. It was pointed out that Dr Trall, a noted physician and author of the late nineteenth century (also considered to be one of the founders of the natural hygiene movement),

> says in his book entitled *Sexual Pathology* that generating children is the main purpose of sexual intercourse between men and women, so that you

> should avoid periods of pregnancy and breast feeding and also avoid the first four days of menstruation; if coitus happens within the next 12 days and if both the young partners are free from diseases, then the woman would conceive.[11]

Polygamy and debauchery were criticized on health grounds. It was pointed out that sexual intercourse with multiple partners, which could be an outcome of polygamy or debauchery, 'makes the bodies of men and women so weak that they can never be healthy and virile again.'[12] Masturbation and nocturnal pollution[13] were identified as two vices which not only weakened the body, but also led 'to a number of serious diseases such as impotence, epilepsy, sex mania, mental imbalance, loss of intelligence, etc.'[14]

A great deal of concern was expressed in different writings regarding the adverse impact of masturbation on the health of adolescent boys and girls. One of the main objections raised against masturbation was that it was aimless, there being no relation between this habit and reproduction; so this habit led only to a deterioration of health. Further, masturbation, through individual physical deterioration, was seen to lead to the social decline of the country and was identified as one of the main causes of India's backwardness. It was pointed out that women who indulged in masturbation became reluctant to face social gatherings. Moreover, 'they have thin bodies, pale faces and sunken eyes with dark circles around them, their heartbeat and their pulse run slow and their bodies emit a kind of bad odour. The sweetness of their voice and behaviour and the beauty of their bodies are gradually lost, and they feel ashamed to look at men.'[15]

Dr Annada Charan Khastagir observed in *A Treatise on the Science and Practice of Midwifery with Diseases of Children and Women*, a textbook written for the students of the Bengali class at the medical school, that

> masturbation by young girls was a cause of hypertrophy of the clitoris. Apparently the practice was common in many schools, and was believed to be addictive and damaging to the brain.... To stop masturbation, the remedy prescribed was a grain of opium and three grains of camphor made into a paste and taken three times daily, as well as the application of ice on the clitoris. The clitoris was medically recognized as the central organ of arousal. To increase desire, an electric current through

the clitoris was recommended, and to decrease it, the clitodorectomy operation; less drastically, a strong caustic lotion or ice could be placed on the clitoris.[16]

In the discursive domain, Indian reformers showed anxious preoccupation with reformulating sexual norms and practices within the household by targeting women. Sometimes it was pointed out that in the *andarmahal* (inner quarters), a lot of female conversation was centred on *adiras* or sexual matters. Women were often criticized for unrefined tastes revealed through crude conversation of a sexual nature. Apparently one of the ways of passing leisure time by women was listening to stories related to sex. According to S.C. Bose women's amusements included needlework, cards, and listening to puerile stories. He even observed, 'Their social tone is neither so pure nor as elevated as becomes a polished, refined community.'[17] Complaints were made about the fact that in such an environment where sex-related matters were openly discussed, little girls became exposed to discussions on sexual matters from such an early stage that they were corrupted.[18]

One alleged source of ill health of women was uncontrolled sexual desire. It was stated:

> Excessive sexual intercourse with one's own husband also breaks a woman's health and changes her behaviour considerably. A wife who used to be gentle in her attitudes and tender in her speech becomes quarrelsome, irate, and short-tempered. Such women stay healthy if they live away from their husbands for a long stretch, but suffer from over bleeding or under-bleeding during menstruation and other diseases when they live with their husbands. This is why men and women are all going to have broken health and short life spans unless they get rid of such unhealthy and harmful habits, and they will never be able to generate healthy and strong children to help the development of the country.[19]

Abinashchandra Kaviratna, the editor of *Chikitsa Sammilani*, wrote:

> Everybody seems to be aware, by virtue of subtle perception or natural intelligence that till the first appearance of menses it is not at all appropriate for girls to have sex with their husbands. Scriptures enjoin this and everyone, wise and foolish alike, is aware of this fact. As it happens, owing to the arousal of sexual desire from close proximity to their husbands,

> girls begin to menstruate and become pregnant at a premature age which causes irreparable damage to the health of the children born of them.[20]

Many popular marriage manuals published during the close of the nineteenth century put emphasis on the regulation of sexuality and the danger and disorder which would result if sexuality was not controlled. In fact, a great deal of emphasis was put on the need to control female sexuality. Some writers argued that it was essential that women should be made aware of their future responsibilities as housewives and mothers through ethical, religious, and practical education since they could not concentrate and think logically like men.[21] Some of the popular manuals, including *Yuvak-yuvati* by Bipradas Mukhopadhyaya (first published in 1891), Yogindranath Mukhopadhyaya's *Jiban Raksa* (1887), and Baradakanta Majumdar's *Naritattva* (1889) went into great detail regarding sexual matters. *Yuvak-yuvati* dealt with subjects like development of the female body, sexual intercourse, pregnancy, birth, and child rearing. It also contained many traditional Hindu rules regarding the times suitable for intercourse and the code of conduct for menstruating women.[22] The widely accepted notion in Bengali society that girls in the company of their husbands were sexually stimulated and thus reached puberty earlier is mentioned here.[23] Baradakanta Majumdar's book, *Naritattva,* expounded reformist views on medical questions regarding consummation of marriage and prescribed that a prolonged period of *gaona,* or the bride's residence at her father's house during the period between marriage and sexual maturity, should be observed so as to delay the onset of the first menses.[24]

The publication of vernacular texts coincided with the publication of official reports which stressed the harmful effects of social customs like child marriage, early consummation of marriage, and so forth. British critics of Bengali sexual practices often blamed child marriage and consummation immediately after puberty for high maternal and infant mortality in Bengal. In 1909, Major W.W. Clemensha, sanitary commissioner of Bengal, pointed out: 'Out of 2700 children that die within the first month [in Calcutta], more than 1200 or nearly 50%, come under the hands of premature birth and debility at birth...probably early marriage is the preponderating factor.'[25] It is interesting to note that apart from sexual matters, domestic practices also became subjects of public discussions.

Domestic Manuals

In nineteenth-century Bengal, reformer–writers produced a large number of Bengali-language domestic manuals. These included manuals addressed simultaneously to men and women, and also included books on health and hygiene and on the rearing of children where the audience intended was unclear. By far the largest number of books included in this collection were advice books written specifically for women—intended to offer them practical and theoretical guidance in family life. Between 1860 and 1900 more than forty advice-for-women manuals were written in Bengali (mostly in the 1880s) and thirty-seven women's magazines and journals came into existence between 1860 and 1910.[26] Whether published as separate books or within the pages of contemporary women's magazines, these works ranged in content from purely medical discussions concerning hygiene and disease, to discussions on household management, housework, child-rearing practices, and cooking, to delineations of family relationships.

These writings sought to disseminate, among other things, knowledge about health, medicine, and diseases. The common perception was that women needed medical guidance since women's ignorance about health norms to be followed would cause harm to the health of family members. It was even pointed out that women who were ignorant of the rules of the body would not only harm themselves, but by producing weak and deficient children would also destroy the nation.[27]

Pratapchandra Majumdar, one of the early authors on the new role of women, remarked, 'Because of the flaws of the mother, the child is ruined; when the child is ruined, the family is ruined; when family life crumbles, society decays; and when society is polluted, no nation can advance.'[28] Educated urban women were assumed to be physically weaker than rural women because they missed the exercise rural women performed while fulfilling their daily household duties.[29]

Women themselves showed concern about the danger posed by uneducated women to the healthy development of children. An anonymous mother pointed out to her daughter:

> Look what dangerous and useless things ignorant women do if their children fall ill.... Sometimes they use *mantras* [words or chants that are believed to have special spiritual powers] to drive the disease away,

> sometimes they perform their own religious rituals. None of these are proper treatments, and do so much harm besides! If they had had a proper education they would not do such ridiculous things.[30]

One way of improving health conditions was for mothers themselves to know something of different hygienic, dietary, and medical principles and apply those to deliver health care. A great deal of pedagogical literature including home manuals and medical and quasi-medical literature published in this period produced a normative discourse on family, included guidelines for proper home management, scientific nurturing of children, regulation of dietary habits, creation of a hygienic environment, and so on. This focus on reformulating domestic habits and norms for improved health constituted part of a new and modern idea of domesticity shared by reform-minded Indians.

In the nineteenth century, the dominance of British power in India imposed an alien culture on the indigenous lifeworlds of the region. From the point of view of the colonized, the presence of colonial modernity as an alternative cultural system problematized all areas of indigenous life. By the last quarter of the nineteenth century, the penetration of colonial culture became very widespread in urban centres such as Calcutta, and every aspect of Hindu domestic life became contested ground. The need to respond to the civilizing mission of colonial ideology and to new conditions of life and work in British India had led Bengali and Indian men to construct new definitions of their own identities and roles, and relationships with the women in their homes. The Hindu woman and her domestic world were at the centre of a debate over colonial modernity and indigenous home and family life.

Colonial modernity had many meanings within late nineteenth-century India. Several scholars have explored its relationship with emerging nationalist discourses, its connections with the revitalization of the Hindu Renaissance, its role in transforming traditions of music and art, and its incompatibilities with indigenous aesthetics.[31] It can also be added that new notions of health, hygiene, and diseases became part of a new ideal of indigenous domesticity through which the indigenous reformers sought to negotiate and reformulate the received notion of colonial modernity (in the arena of health practices). These ideas of health and hygiene were an integral part of a new idea of colonial domesticity.

Domesticity

The secular discourse of domesticity, which essentially meant a set of ideas about the proper ordering of home and family relations, was produced originally in Europe.[32] This domestic discourse was centred round the conviction that the 'natural' order of human relations involved a patriarchal family system with a gendered separation of spheres of activity and the husband at the head of the family unit.[33] System, order, and efficiency were regarded as essential components of daily domestic life. It was also believed that a proper ordering of home and family life would come from the application of science and scientific methods to the domestic sphere. At the same time, the ambitious nineteenth-century European bourgeois classes wished to see themselves as universally hegemonic, which eventually led them to promote domesticity (as well as reason, citizenship, and market economics) as a natural and universal category of human life.[34]

Bourgeois domestic discourse and the practices rising from it were gradually incorporated into the civilizing mission of colonialism itself.[35] In India, colonial administrators, to buttress their own legitimacy, disparaged the miserable conditions of women. Indian ideas of domestic life were described as 'barbaric' and demeaning for women, when compared to Europe's 'civilized' notions about domesticity in general, and women's freedom and equality in particular. In his *The History of British India* (1826), James Mill stated: 'Nothing can exceed the habitual contempt which the Hindus entertain for their women. [They]...are held...in extreme degradation.'[36]

The English-educated Indians in the city of Calcutta (mostly high-caste Hindus), as in other parts of India, had access to all the discourses of British colonial modernity and the 'civilizing mission', and to colonialism's negative formulations of Indian identity and culture as 'decadent', 'weak', and 'effeminate'.

To colonial critique of Indian domestic practices (including women's supposed inferior position) and to changing demand of life under British rule, English-educated and Western-influenced Indian men responded by focusing on the need to reform women's social conditions, most particularly women's literacy and education, which they saw as the key to both India's progress and their own. The main social utility of women's educational project was seen as lying in the constructive role expected to be played by the new women in bringing about moral and social welfare of family members.[37] Bengali male intelligentsia's social reform programme centring around the women's question in the nineteenth century was shaped to a large extent by the need of reformulating norms and functions of middle-class family life as a site of moral and cultural restructuring of the nation. The issue of education, in a way, formed the core area in the agenda of reforming women's conditions, and women's education had little to do with economic functions or pursuit of employment, growth of professional expertise, and so forth.

In the colonial situation, most English-educated bhadralok were subjected to humiliation in their working lives and 'they required the type of wife who could provide sympathetic care and create the atmosphere of a peaceful haven in their own homes'.[38] Women were to be intelligent companions for the emergent bhadralok. It was thought that in a marriage between an educated and an illiterate girl, discord and disagreement were bound to arise. The Western-educated elite section of the society, imbued with liberal ideas, sought educated wives as companions or 'helpmates'.[39] From the 1860s, it became a practice for men to travel to different postings with their wives. It was contrary to the traditional notion of the wife's domestic role and to the concept of the traditional joint family.[40] The younger, educated generation was no longer willing to marry uneducated girls. In an essay titled 'Strisiksha' in *Jnanankur* in the 1870s, it was argued that women of upper- and middle-class Hindu society had to be imparted some education in order to find a bridegroom. These new educated women were expected to develop as companions to men, as scientific nurturers, and as members of civil society; they were to remain a socially distanced class from the common or lower-class women who inhabited a world of unrefined, coarse, popular culture.[41]

It has been pointed out that the nationalist reformers of this period offered women participation in a 'new patriarchy'.[42] Older indigenous patriarchal traditions had demanded that women remain illiterate and uneducated, confined to the home's inner quarters, the antahpur. Colonially modern Indian men imagined a new order that although facilitated women's literacy and education, also maintained that women would remain in a dependent and subordinate status within

Indian society. It has been asserted that Hindu nationalists who were excluded from the political power structure of the British Raj came to define the domestic world as their own—outside the purview of colonial intervention. This was to be the private domain of the nation over which they could achieve some measure of mastery and autonomous self-identification. Thus, Partha Chatterjee has argued, long before the nationalists began their political struggle with British imperialism, they had produced a domain of sovereignty within colonial society itself, a domain that included the domestic world of women and the family.[43] The 'new woman' of nationalist construction was to inculcate in herself 'the virtues—the typically bourgeois virtues characteristic of the new social norms of "disciplining"—of orderliness, thrift, cleanliness, and a personal sense of responsibility, the practical skills of literacy, accounting, hygiene, and the ability to run the household according to the new physical and economic conditions set by the outside world'.[44] Punctuality, cleanliness, order, and discipline were seen as the inherent characteristics of modern European homes; dirt, disorder, and disease characterized the indigenous household.[45]

A large number of pedagogical texts written by reformers in this period, which produced a normative discourse on family, included guidelines for an ideal housewife for proper home management, scientific nurturing of children, regulation of dietary habits, creation of hygienic environment, and so forth. Many studies have explored the social reforms and the gender relations of late nineteenth-century India, revealing the inherently patriarchal nature of both, and often, patriarchy's triumph as social reform was 'resolved' (that is to say, abandoned) in the growing nationalist fervour at the turn of the century. It can be argued, following Judith Walsh, that the new patriarchy that produced domestic literatures, challenged—in addition to the ideas and customs of an older Hindu patriarchy—the power and authority of the extended family. The husband's claim to authority over the wife was asserted over and against the existing power and control of family elders, particularly the family's older women, who were considered as barriers to reforms. The authority of elderly women was sought to be replaced by that of the Western-educated, colonial, modern husband.[46]

The Reading Woman

It has been argued by Benedict Anderson that print literature (along with the print capitalists who produced it) was of particular importance to nineteenth-century bourgeoisies, the middle classes of Europe and the Americas. It is through print, Anderson argues, that these middle classes came to imagine their mutual existence.[47] In colonial India, too, the nineteenth-century discourse on domesticity was produced in the world of print and was consumed naturally by literate members of society. By the mid-nineteenth century, a substantial publishing industry had developed in urban centres of the British Raj. In Bengal, the publication of Bengali-language books had become an income-producing activity for many. The growth of a class of educated girls also created demand for books in print. Over the nineteenth century, the number of girls attending schools continued to rise. In 1862–3, the government's report on public instruction published its first statistics on women's educational institutions in Bengal. It recorded the existence of 15 schools for girls and 530 attending students.[48] By 1881, government reports for Bengal listed the number of women's schools at 1,042 and of girl students at 44,096. By 1891, the number of schools had doubled to 2,239 and the number of students had risen to 78,865.[49] Newly literate women needed new reading materials. 'The first manuals for women appeared in the 1860s just as the schools for girls became statistically visible. Over the rest of the century, the number of manuals increased along with (and as a result of) the growth of girls' literacy and of women's schools throughout the province.'[50]

In the 1860s and 1870s, home education (the zenana system) and home tutoring were the preferred methods of educating women, and Bengali writers initially produced advice literature for girls keeping this in mind. Zenana education was promoted by European female missionaries who were employed by educated families to give private tuition to the female members. Home education or instruction provided by male members of the family to the female members was a scheme that was adopted more frequently. Home education and zenana education were accepted by those who did not desire to break purdah restrictions by sending girls to schools. Despite some disadvantages, homeschooling remained popular at least till the end of the nineteenth century.[51] Between 1880 and 1900, the publication of domestic manuals surged and more than forty advice-for-women books were brought into print (by the Bengal Library, between 1879 and 1896). A large number of these writings dealt with health care advice for women. Many domestic manuals taught details of hygiene, nursing, home remedies, child-rearing, and so on. Health advice to women, aiming at modernizing the family, became an integral part of the new ideal of domesticity. Women had to play a crucial and far more important role than before in this standardized, reformulated style of domesticity. With the emergence of the family as a site where nationalist restructuring was to be carried out, women were awarded a special, augmented status in remodelling the private domain of the nation. The bhadramahila was expected to master the technique of becoming a *sugrihini* (adept homemaker) by acquiring elementary knowledge of all sorts of medical remedies—allopathy, homeopathy, kabiraji, as well as unani or hakimi—for treating at least the common ailments to save the family a lot of expense in doctors' fees.[52] Allopathic treatment was criticized by some for its harmful side effects and too much dependence on this kind of treatment was assumed to be an outcome of women's loss of knowledge regarding local herbal remedies. Women were often criticized for having lost the expertise in native folk medicine, held by women of previous generations, and for harming children by giving them Western medicine. Rajnarain Bose, for example, pointed out that children of recent generations were weaker than in the past because their mothers treated them with Western rather than native medicines.[53] Childcare manuals aimed at modernizing child-rearing practices in Bengali families mostly emphasized the need of following a regular routine in matters of the infants' breastfeeding and also spacing of the diet to be delivered to a child.[54]

Ramanir Kartavya (Duties of Women, 1890), composed by the two authors Giribala Mitra and Jayakrishna Mitra, contained sections on child-rearing where readers would learn what to feed a baby from infancy up to two years of age. It included general advice on which food items were nutritious and also pointed out that every room of a house should be regularly and thoroughly cleaned for cleanliness to improve everyone's health.[55]

Satyacharan Mitra, in his book *Strir prati svamir upades* (A Husband's Advice to His Wife), wrote about the benefits of using neem twigs instead of tooth powder for cleaning teeth.[56] Various women's magazines also published health advice to impart knowledge to women. In a number of writings, emphasis was put on the necessity of a sense of cleanliness, hygienic environment, and fresh air for the protection of health and prevention of diseases. It was even pointed out that an indispensable part of *garhyasthya dharma* (household duties and responsibilities to be imparted by a married person) and the compulsory domestic acts to be performed by a Hindu female consisted of cleaning and washing bed linen, dusting twice daily, and purifying drinking water.[57] Sometimes social customs like the purdah system, early motherhood, and so on, were linked to adverse health conditions by women themselves. *Bamabodhini Patrika* (the longest surviving women's magazine covering a period of almost sixty years from 1863 to 1922), published from 1871 onwards, carried a regular feature on elementary home remedies, called 'Garhasthya cikitsa pranali' (domestic treatment regime).[58] In a section titled 'Panchan O Mushtijog' the magazine provided advice to deal with various health hazards without consulting a doctor. *Bamabodhini* introduced a new section entitled 'upadesher jhuri' (basket of advice) in the 1920s, where advice was given to the housewife about various health hazards and hygienic problems associated with housework and cooking.

Another magazine titled *Mahila*, in a serialized section titled 'Akasmik Ghatana o Samanya Rogidiger Griha Chikitsa', imparted advice regarding elementary measures to be taken in case of sudden accidental illnesses. Women readers were often advised about the essential needs of purified water, unpolluted air, and healthy diet required to lead healthy family lives. Sometimes herbal home remedies were prescribed and indigenous alternative therapies and Western remedies were suggested simultaneously. One reason for the advocacy and popularization of local remedies was their cheapness. At the same time, middle-class Indians were not averse to adopting Western medical knowledge because it was considered to be the vehicle of progress. As pointed out by Borthwick, women had to learn at least the rudiments of Western medical treatment.[59] Women themselves were becoming aware of the importance of acquiring at least some basic knowledge of the different forms of therapies and supported that. For example, one female writer advocated the 'common-sense' observance of certain rules of hygiene along with the use of Western drugs.[60]

With the institutionalization of medicine in the nineteenth century and the emergence and spread of the knowledge of a group of professional doctors, more and more families were becoming exposed to various kinds of expertise on medical matters, child-rearing, and other such subjects. Parents were advised to follow the dictates of experts and to prepare themselves by reading appropriate books and journals. Doctors themselves wrote health primers for women. Parents, especially mothers, were expected to become the experts' allies, the supposed educators of the family, and executors of the experts' orders. Instructions like the following, for instance, were quite common: 'For the proper rearing of children, for proper knowledge about the child's nutrition and health, you should read appropriate books, you should take advice from expert physicians.'[61] As pointed out here, we see an emphasis on an outside authority—medical experts or qualified doctors. In the new situation, mothers were expected to educate themselves to be able to understand and execute the medical experts' instructions to which the family had become exposed.

At the same time, they were expected to act as a repository of traditional knowledge. Women, in their capacity as mothers, were to play a central role in national health regeneration through their influence over hygienic conditions within the household, and also by understanding that professional medicine was supposed to act as the best guarantee of health in complicated situations. The responsible mother was one who made provision in the household budget for a physician's care. Women no doubt continued to act as their families' primary caregivers. Sick people were still more likely to be treated at home than in a hospital, and even if they consulted a doctor at his clinic, they only had brief contact with him. Sickness could arise at any moment and in any place, whereas it was impossible for the physician to be everywhere at all times. Hence, medical professionals relied upon the assistance of women who could, it was assumed, offer more constant care to sick family members. As mothers were most often the ones who cared for the entire family's health, physicians knew that if they were to expand their clientele, their best hope for reaching patients within a family was to gain the confidence of the mothers. Advertisements for doctors and medicines that aimed at women as the main consumers were published in different journals; the products advertised included patent medicines, kabiraji as well as homeopathic medicines prepared by physicians as well as pharmaceutical companies.

Most doctors considered that if women were to be entrusted with the duty to ensure that proper medical treatments were administered, their education must eliminate any remnants of folk medical traditions or popular 'superstitions'. Girls were warned that listening to traditional sources of advice, especially older women, was foolish and dangerous. It was common to associate the figure of the older woman with superstition and error and thus to discredit her as a source of medical advice. The exhortation to respect the doctor's authority over healing was, however, not entirely free of tension. Although home manuals repeatedly asserted that young women should aspire to be good assistants to the physician, the majority of the pages devoted to lessons on basic medical care, nonetheless, focused on developing a woman's own skills and know-how in order to prepare her to treat numerous common ailments. The emphasis was, therefore, implicitly on training future mothers to be competent caregivers in their own right, and there was no guarantee that women would not simply dispense with the physician in all but dire cases. Home manuals and other didactic writings thus imposed a dual responsibility on women for their families' health: a woman should be competent enough to provide care herself, yet at the same time should entrust the care of her family's health to a physician. In the first case, women were expected to fulfil a role that they had long held in different households: that of the producers of medical care. It was in the second case that women's traditional role of the family's caregiver was subtly redefined to that of consumers of professional medical advice and treatment.

***

The lessons on basic family health care were ultimately a double-edged sword. Although they promoted the virtues of physician-centred health care to a far broader segment of the population than doctors could have hoped to reach in previous centuries, they also preached that a woman should 'be prepared', and in so doing they encouraged readers to purchase remedies that would be useful to have on hand. Medical science had made tremendous advances by the turn of the twentieth century, but general practitioners still relied heavily on the informal assistance of a patient's (usually female) relatives when it came to administering treatment. In this respect, altering women's practices with respect to family health care was an important step in the professionalization of medicine, yet this was not accomplished by simply proclaiming the authority of the 'man of science'. Women also exercised influence over the household budget, and if they were to be persuaded to set aside money for professional medical care, they also had to be approached as consumers.

The dual lesson, that women should know how to consume medical care as well as provide basic treatment themselves, reveals a dimension of the professionalization of medicine that is often overlooked. The emphasis that was placed on deferring to a doctor's judgement greatly resembles efforts to subordinate the activities of untrained professionals to their (the doctors') authority. However, women and their families were also a doctor's potential clients, which complicated any efforts to subordinate women's influence over family health care to the doctor's authority. An essential step in the expansion of the doctors' authority over healing was the renegotiation of women's roles as guardians of their family's health. In this respect, the professionalization of medicine involved educating women as medical consumers.

It may be pointed out that the heterogeneous nature of health advice, contained in domestic manuals as well as in articles published in different periodicals addressed to women, helps us understand the contested medical world which influenced the new world of domesticity. The educated middle class, or the bhadralok as well as the bhadramahila in colonial India, tried to blend indigenous tradition with modern or Western medicine in a bid to reformulate the Western ideal of domesticity.

As pointed out by researchers, biographical evidence shows that some women did try to follow the advice given in the manuals. However, there is no direct evidence that can prove conclusively that the kind of knowledge disseminated actually filtered down to the majority of bhadramahila. The value of these manuals and other writings lies in the fact that they reflect the attitudes of the writers.

As already pointed out, the family was becoming exposed to many outside forces, including the intervention of doctors or trained professional experts, and educated women were expected to assist them; advice contained in manuals and other writings were partly intended to enable them to follow and execute the advice of medical experts.

Theoretically at least, this created the possibility of augmentation of women's power through self-improvement and through acting under the guidance of outside experts, along with the development of their own skills by acquiring some degree of all available forms of elementary medical knowledge. The new, modern, educated woman, by simultaneously absorbing new health guidelines and knowledge of hygiene and treatment and by also acting as the repository of traditional knowledge, would create the possibility of women's empowerment. As modern educated women, they would also understand when the help of a doctor was needed. In the emerging overall socio-medical rhetoric of degeneration, biomedical issues and socio-cultural norms were conflated and the vitality of the individual and the national body was closely linked. If the health of the nation depended upon the health of the individual bodies, then personal health could not remain a purely private matter. By this reasoning, reform-minded educated elites (and physicians) tended to hold the view that it was in the best interest of individuals and the nation to preserve health through dissemination of knowledge about health preservation, by adopting rational, scientific, and hygienic measures and by entrusting the treatment of different acute illnesses to medical professionals.

Manuals and prescriptive literature reveal that the Bengali bhadralok's constructions of the moral universe were centred on the home and the family and that it reinforced caste, class, and gender boundaries through the hierarchical, dependent, power relationships in colonial households. The ideological drive to prescribe a code of behaviour for the sugrihini or the *adarsha mata* (ideal mother) reflected not only the middle-class attempt to define its own cultural identity, but also its engagement in an ideological struggle to come to grips with the twin pressures of colonialism and nationalism. The prescriptive discourse of the ideologues and reformers that developed around middle-class women in general betrayed a tension that was deeply implicated in contested notions of tradition, modernity, and the nation—particularly noticeable in the advice for the adoption of new health principles as well as for not ignoring old practices altogether. New principles of hygiene can also be interpreted as seeking to reinforce caste, class, and gender boundaries and thus contributed to the new cultural construction of middle-class identity as separate and distinct from the lower classes and castes.

By the end of the nineteenth century, the new discourse on sexuality and domesticity that was aimed at refashioning the private domain coincided with important social/marriage reform debates like the one aroused by the proposed Age of Consent Bill of 1891. The Act has been interpreted as an important British challenge to the control exerted by Bengali men over female sexuality.[62] There was the convergence of medical opinion and nationalist agitation over raising the age of permissible sexual intercourse in marriage from ten to twelve. In the first Age of Consent debate of 1891, women's organizations were ultimately successful in persuading Lansdowne, the viceroy, and Scoble, the legal member of the viceroy's council, of the need for legal intervention in early marriages despite anticipated opposition from revivalists and the orthodoxy. The Arya Mahila Samaj, a pioneering women's organization created by Pandita Ramabai in Maharashtra, was active in persuading British lady doctors in India to send a strong petition graphically describing the physical injuries due to early cohabitation of thirteen girl-brides whom they encountered in the course of their careers. The Arya Mahila Samaj also enlisted the support of Dr Edith Pechey, an outspoken medical critic of early marriages, in their public meetings and petitions. The importance of medical evidence in this contentious debate was underlined by the frequency with which petitioners referred to early marriages as a major cause of the declining physiques of Indians. Numerous petitions from physicians in Bengal were included in the legislative proceedings, as was also an extract from Chever's medical jurisprudence on the damaging physiological and psychological consequences for women of early consummation and early maternity.

The controversy surrounding the Age of Consent Act of 1891 represented the first time that reformers had successfully used allopathic medical arguments in an issue of social reforms for women. It indicated the extent to which women's bodies had become politicized by the 1890s and how it could influence legal debate.

In the first half of the twentieth century, arguments of biomedicine continued to dominate imperial discourse and practice of medical intervention to even greater extents. Debates regarding marriage reform and demographic considerations, controversies regarding birth-control measures, and linking of the question of Indian (men's and) women's health to imperial neglect flooded the public sphere and dominated the issues regarding women and medicine.

Notes and References

1. See articles like 'Indigenous Health Science', *Swasthya*, Magh, B.S. 1307 (January–February 1901). Cited in Pradip Kumar Bose, ed., *Health and Society in Bengal: A Selection from Late 19th-Century Bengali Periodicals* (New Delhi: SAGE Publications, 2006), pp. 126–38; 'Precepts for Good Health', *Vigyan Darpan*, Bhadra, B.S. 1289 (August–September 1882). Cited in Bose, *Health and Society in Bengal*, pp. 120–2; 'The Revival of National Physical Health', *Chikitsa Sammilani*, Baisakh, B.S. 1292 (April–May 1885). Cited in P. Bose, *Health and Society in Bengal*, pp. 105–16.

2. *Chikitsa Sammilani* (Baisakh, B.S. 1292) (April–May 1885), cited in P. Bose, *Health and Society in Bengal*, p. 105.

3. 'The Revival of National Physical Health', *Chikitsa Sammilani*, Baisakh B.S. 1292 (April–May 1885). Cited in P. Bose, *Health and Society in Bengal*, pp. 101–16, especially p. 105.

4. See David Arnold, *The New Cambridge History of India*, vol. 3, part 5, *Science, Technology and Medicine in Colonial India* (Cambridge: University Press, 2000), pp. 75–81.

5. 'The Revival of National Physical Health'. Cited in P. Bose, *Health and Society in Bengal*, p. 106.

6. 'The Revival of National Physical Health'. Cited in P. Bose, *Health and Society in Bengal*, p. 106.

7. 'National Health—How Marriage Affects It', Swastha, Magh, B.S. 1307 (January–February 1901). Cited in P. Bose, *Health and Society in Bengal*, p. 138.

8. 'National Health—How Marriage Affects It'. Cited in P. Bose, *Health and Society in Bengal*, p. 134.

9. Suryanarayan Ghosh, *Baigyanik Dampatya Pranali* (Dhaka: 1884), p. 32.

10. 'The Revival of National Physical Health'. Cited in P. Bose, *Health and Society in Bengal*, p. 111.

11. 'The Revival of National Physical Health'. Cited in P. Bose, *Health and Society in Bengal*, p. 113.

12. 'The Revival of National Physical Health'. Cited in Bose, *Health and Society in Bengal*, p. 107.

13. 'Having an ejaculation while sleeping is known as nocturnal pollution.' See 'The Revival of National Physical Health'. Cited in P. Bose, *Health and Society in Bengal*, p. 109.

15. 'The Revival of National Physical Health'. Cited in P. Bose, *Health and Society in Bengal*, p. 110.

16. Annada Charan Khastagir, *A Treatise on the Science and Practice of Midwifery with Diseases of Children and Women: Manabjanmatattwa, dhatri*

bidya, nabaprasuta sisu o strijatir byadhisangraha, 2nd ed. (Calcutta: 1878 [1868]), pp. 624–5. Also cited in Meredith Borthwick, *The Changing Role of Women in Bengal: 1849–1905* (Princeton, New Jersey: Princeton University Press, 1984), pp. 135–6.

17. S.C. Bose, *The Hindoos as They Are: A Description of the Manners, Customs and Inner Life of Hindu Society in Bengal* (Calcutta: 1881), p. 8. Also cited in Borthwick, *The Changing Role of Women in Bengal*, p. 19.

18. See Borthwick, *The Changing Role of Women in Bengal*, pp. 18–19.

19. 'The Revival of National Physical Health'. Cited in P. Bose, *Health and Society in Bengal*, p. 110.

20. P. Bose, *Health and Society in Bengal*, p. 152.

21. Baradakanta Majumdar, *Naritattva* (Calcutta: 1889), pp. 30–5. Also cited in Dagmar Engels, *Beyond Purdah? Women in Bengal 1890–1939* (New Delhi: Oxford University Press, 1996), p. 83.

22. Bipradas Mukhopadhyaya, *Yuvak-yuvati* (Calcutta: 1922 [1891]), pp. 42–51. Also cited in Engels, *Beyond Purdah? Women in Bengal*, p. 82.

23. B. Mukhopadhyaya, *Yuvak-yuvati*, p. 42.

24. B. Majumdar, *Naritattva*, pp. 40–1. Also cited in Engels, *Beyond Purdah? Women in Bengal*, p. 83.

25. *Census of India*, 1911, vol. 6, part I, p. 31.

26. Usha Chakraborty, *Conditions of Bengali Women around the 2nd Half of the 19th Century* (Calcutta: Self-published, 1963), pp. 184–5, 190–1.

27. Prasannatara Gupta, *Paribarikjiban* (Calcutta: Kuntaleen Press, 1903), p. 82. Cited in Pradip Kumar Bose, 'Sons of the Nation: Child Rearing in the New Family', *Texts of Power: Emerging Disciplines in Colonial Bengal*, edited by Partha Chatterjee (Calcutta: Samya, 1996), p. 123.

28. Pratapchandra Majumdar, *Stricharitra* (Calcutta: Nababidhan, 1891), p. 14; cited in P. Bose, 'Sons of the Nation', p. 123.

29. Dineschandra Sen, *Grihasri* (Calcutta: 1915), p. 134. Also cited in Engels, *Beyond Purdah? Women in Bengal*, p. 82.

30. 'Kanyar prati matar dvitiya upades', *Bamabodhini Patrika* 1, no. 2 (1864). Cited in Borthwick, *The Changing Role of Women in Bengal*, p. 65.

31. See, for example, works like the following: Partha Chatterjee, *Nationalist Thought and the Colonial World* (Minneapolis: University of Minnesota Press, 1986); Partha Chatterjee, 'The Nationalist Resolution of the Women's Question' in *Recasting Women: Essays in Colonial History*, edited by Kumkum Sangari and Sudesh Vaid (New Brunswick: Rutgers University Press, 1990); Partha Chatterjee, *The Nation and Its Fragments: Colonial and Postcolonial Histories* (Princeton, New Jersey: Princeton University Press, 1993); Sumit Sarkar, *Writing Social History* (New Delhi: Oxford University Press, 1997); Tanika Sarkar,

Words to Win: The Making of Amar Jiban, a Modern Autobiography (New Delhi: Kali for Women, 1999); Tanika Sarkar, *Hindu Wife, Hindu Nation: Community, Religion, and Cultural Nationalism* (Bloomington: Indiana University Press, 2001); Lakshmi Subramaniam, 'The Master, Muse, and the Nation', *South Asia* 23, no. 2 (2000): 1–32; Brian Hatcher, *Idioms of Improvement: Vidyasagar and Cultural Encounter in Bengal, Delhi* (New Delhi: Oxford University Press, 1996); Dipesh Chakrabarty, *Provincializing Europe: Postcolonial Thought and Historical Difference* (Princeton, New Jersey: Princeton University Press, 2000).

32. Most contemporary scholarship links it with the beginnings of industrialization, industrial capitalism, and the new modes of production of the late eighteenth and early nineteenth centuries. See Carmen Luke, *Pedagogy, Printing and Protestantism: The Discourse on Childhood* (Albany: State University of New York Press, 1989); Leonore Davidoff and Catherine Hall, *Family Fortunes: Men and Women of the English Middle Class, 1780–1850* (Chicago: University of Chicago Press, 1987); Jean Comaroff and John L. Comaroff, 'Home-made Hegemony: Modernity, Domesticity, and Colonialism in South Africa', in *African Encounters with Domesticity*, edited by K. Hansen (New Brunswick: Rutgers University Press, 1992).

33. Davidoff and Hall, *Family Fortunes*.

34. The Comaroffs argue that far from being a universal standard for human family life, nineteenth-century European middle-class domesticity is a discourse and argument marshalled by particular European classes at a particular historical moment, to advance their own claims of cultural hegemony. Comaroff and Comaroff, 'Home-made Hegemony', p. 39.

35. Comaroff and Comaroff, 'Home-made Hegemony'.

36. Quoted in Geraldine Forbes, 'Negotiating Modernities: The Public and Private Worlds of Dr. Haimabati Sen', in *Rhetoric and Reality: Gender and the Colonial Experience in South Asia*, edited by Avril A. Powell and Siobhan Lambert-Hurley (New Delhi: Oxford University Press, 2006), p. 225.

37. Himani Bannerji, 'Fashioning a Self: Educational Proposals For and By Women in Popular Magazines in Colonial Bengal', *Economic and Political Weekly* 26, no. 43 (1991): 38. Borthwick, *The Changing Role of Women in Bengal*, p. 116.

39. Borthwick, *The Changing Role of Women in Bengal*, pp. 114–24.

40. Borthwick, *The Changing Role of Women in Bengal*, p. 48.

41. Forbes, *The New Cambridge History of India*, vol. 4, part 2, *Women in Modern India*, p. 41. Also see Sumanta Banerjee, 'Marginalization of Women's Popular Culture in Nineteenth Century Bengal', in Sangari and Vaid, *Recasting Women*, pp. 127–79.

42. P. Chatterjee, *Nationalist Thought and the Colonial World*; P. Chatterjee, *The Nation and Its Fragments*.

43. P. Chatterjee, *The Nation and Its Fragments*, p. 6.

44. P. Chatterjee, *The Nation and Its Fragments*, pp. 129–30.

45. Dipesh Chakrabarty, 'Postcoloniality and the Artifice of History', in *A Subaltern Studies Reader: 1986–1995*, edited by Ranajit Guha (Minneapolis: University of Minnesota Press, 1997), p. 277.

46. See Judith E. Walsh, *How to Be The Goddess of Your Home: An Anthology of Bengali Domestic Manuals* (New Delhi: Yoda Press, 2005).

47. See Benedict Anderson, *Imagined Communities: Reflections on the Origin and Spread of Nationalism*, revised and extended edition (London: Verso, 1991).

48. Jogesh C. Bagal, 'History of Bethune School and College: 1849–1949', in *Bethune School & College Centenary Volume, 1849–1949*, edited by Kalidas Nag (Calcutta: S.N. Guha Ray, 1949), p. 25; U. Chakraborty, *Conditions of Bengali Women*, p. 47.

49. Ghulam Murshid, *Reluctant Debutante: Response of Bengali Women to Modernization, 1849–1905* (Rajshahi: Rajshahi University Press, 1983), p. 43.

50. Judith E. Walsh, *Domesticity in Colonial India: What Women Learned When Men Gave Them Advice* (New Delhi: Oxford university Press, 2004).

51. Murshid, *Reluctant Debutante*, p. 43.

52. In 1878, a native doctor's fee varied from Rs 3 to Rs 10; a European doctor charged Rs 16. Lady Doctors charged Rs 10 per visit. Borthwick, *The Changing Role of Women in Bengal*, p. 217.

53. Rajnarain Bose, *Se Kal ar E Kal* (Calcutta: Chirayet, 1976 [1874]), p. 87. Also cited in Borthwick, *The Changing Role of Women in Bengal*, p. 220.

54. Borthwick, *The Changing Role of Women in Bengal*, pp. 170–8.

55. Walsh, *How to Be the Goddess of Your Home*.

56. It was published in Calcutta in 1884. He wrote at least eight books in his lifetime. Four were works of fiction. Among his seven Bengali books, four focused on women. *A Husband's Advice to His Wife* was self-published. The following is an extract from Chapter 8, titled 'The Daily Activities of Women', of the book.

> Husband (H): You should clean your teeth with coal powder. Or, if you use a neem twig or a twig from an asheora tree, that would be even better.
>
> Wife (W): Girls should be using twigs to clean their teeth! Is that what you are saying?
>
> H: When you clean your teeth, if you do use a tooth twig, it keeps your teeth in good condition, hardens their outsides and rids your mouth of odour—so everyone, man or woman, should clean his or her teeth in this way...

> W: But where could I get such a twig in the city every day?
>
> H: If a twig isn't available you should clean your teeth with coal powder. But if a tooth twig could be obtained (from a neem or an asheora tree) that would be a great deal better. These days the state of Bengali Babus is such that they cannot understand the benefits of tooth twigs. They do not understand how beneficial neem or asheora twigs are for the teeth—instead they only agitate for 'tooth powder' 'tooth powder'.

(Translation from Walsh, *Domesticity in Colonial India.*)
Also see Walsh, *How to Be the Goddess of Your Home.*

57. 'Narir kartabya', *Bamabodhini Patrika* 2, no. 3 (May 1881): 196; Kumudini Ray, 'Hindu narir garhasthya dharmma', *Bamabodhini Patrika* 5, no. 3 (December 1894): 359; 'Swasthya raksa', *Bamabodhini Patrika* 2, no. 2 (September 1880): 188. Also cited in Borthwick, *The Changing Role of Women in Bengal*, p. 207.

58. *Bamabodhini Patrika* 8: 100, (December 1871). Also cited in Borthwick, *The Changing Role of Women in Bengal*, p. 219.

59. Borthwick, *The Changing Role of Women in Bengal*, p. 220.

60. Lilabati Mitra, 'Grihaswasthye ramanir dristi', *Antahpur* 7: 9. Also cited in Borthwick, *The Changing Role of Women in Bengal*, p. 221.

61. P. Bose, 'Sons of the Nation', p. 123.

62. See Engels, *Beyond Purdah? Women in Bengal.*

5 *Women's Work and the Politics of Health*

During the first half of the twentieth century, Indian society witnessed many crucial developments, including the intensification of the nationalist struggle, heightened discussion on the growth and development of the Indian nation, and increasing colonial onslaught on Indian social practices by the imperialists. As pointed out by many, the 'heady and tumultuous decades' of the 1920s and the 1930s saw the imperial public spheres saturated with the 'woman question.'[1] It has been argued that during the twentieth century, issues of the 'private domain' were neither repressed, nor resolved, nor absent from public sphere debates in colonial India;[2] rather, this period experienced heightened public interest and veritable discourses on the body and sexuality. These discourses reflected the anxieties of late nineteenth-century social reformers, who had drawn attention towards the need to build stronger, masculine bodies, and the increasing involvement of nationalist Indians in the search for ways of building up a strong, robust nation.[3] Maternal and child welfare, demographic reform, and national strength were regarded as constitutive features of modern public health sensibilities—which would link welfare of the individual body to the emergence of a strong nation. Alongside, birth control and eugenics—supported by international efforts and initiatives of private Indians—became objects of immense attention.[4]

Moreover, as the Montagu–Chelmsford Reforms (1919) made health a provincial responsibility, some amount of government effort was noticeable in the field of organizing health education for mothers and children. Another notable and unprecedented development noticed in the early twentieth century was the increasing participation of women themselves in the arena of health welfare—the result of a gradual rise in the number of women medical personnel, emergence of women's organizations, and the rising involvement of imperial women in philanthropic activities.

Imperial Initiatives

Apart from the curative practice of hospital medicine, intrusive health education for mother and children, organization of baby shows, and publicity and sale of medical literature became new features of colonial public health initiatives in the early twentieth century. As has been pointed out, 'After an earlier focus on the medicalization of childbirth which sought to provide scientific training for midwives and to establish facilities such as maternity hospitals with specialized obstetricians, the emphasis was now shifting to the extension of ante and post natal care to mothers and children.'[5]

The concern for public health, and infant and maternal mortality was not restricted to India, but was in fact a global phenomenon. In the changing international scenario of the early twentieth century, improvements in maternal and infant health became matters of worldwide interest. Increasing imperial rivalries and anxieties about the future health condition of the children of the armymen, to some extent, prompted certain measures aimed at improving the health of mothers and children. England witnessed a steep downward trend in infant mortality between 1903 and 1908. According to scholars, these years of transition coincided with 'the real take-off of the health visiting movement, and it is reasonable to conclude that the movement did have a sizeable impact on the infant death rate'.[6] High rates of sickness amongst British soldiers during the Boer War pointed out the necessity of adopting health measures to lessen infant mortality and diseases among the working class (since most of the army recruits belonged to this class) in order to increase the efficiency of the troops and workforce in the face of steep international conflicts. Anna Davin, in her essay 'Imperialism and Motherhood', has analysed the increasing British interest in the politics of birth and childcare during the first decades of the twentieth century. In post–World War I Britain, the activities culminated in the 1918 Maternity and Child Welfare Act, 'which envisaged the provision of a network of infant welfare centres'.[7]

The twentieth century also witnessed the growing importance of personal or individual hygiene in place of older ideas of macro-sanitation and public hygiene in public health measures. While in the older model individuals were considered as irrational beings incapable of inculcating healthy domestic practices or pursuing elevated standards of personal or domestic habits, in the twentieth century, a strong effort was made towards individual health education for improving personal hygiene. One important fallout of this hygienic model was the increased influence of eugenics societies, which put stress on biological fitness and purity of race. Women's roles as natural biological reproducers and conscious mothers of healthy children were emphasized immensely. Thus the expansion of the middle-class family ideal, with the mother as the homemaker and father as the provider, was at the core of public health projects in the early years of the twentieth century, including the Child Welfare Movement.[8]

The infant death rate in England around 1870 was 162. It came down to 96 in 1917 and in 1920, it was as low as 80 per 1,000. In contrast, during the first two decades of the twentieth century in Bengal, one in five babies died before the first birthday. In many of the large towns in England, the infant death rate was below seventy in 1919, and in some of the smaller towns, even below fifty. In contrast to this, it was found that in India 'there is scarcely a large town in which the infant mortality rate is not higher than 200 and in many of the largest towns it is more than 400'.[9]

In India, maternal health condition came under the close scrutiny of colonial observers, particularly women medical professionals, in the early twentieth century. Journalist Mary Frances Billington, who made a trip to India, wrote in the 1890s that infant mortality was very high in India. However (as pointed out by David Arnold), though rates of maternal mortality were believed to be very high during the first half of the twentieth century, there was little reliable statistical evidence to prove it or to establish its cause, characteristics, and social distribution.[10] Members of the Women's Medical Service (WMS) showed their interest in investigating the problems related to women's health.[11] Dagmar Curjel, in an essay titled 'Improvement of the Conditions of Childbirth in India', pointed out that miscarriages, abortions, and stillbirths accounted for 34 per cent of pregnancies while the survival rate among infants seemed to be 49 per cent.[12] In Calcutta, female mortality rate was reported to be over 5 per cent whereas the rate of male mortality was over 3.3 per cent. The difference seemed to be the sharpest when compared between men and women in the age group of fifteen to forty years.[13] In 1921, infant mortality rates were still on the increase and were, even among the bhadralok, double the corresponding proportions in European countries.[14] In 1940, infant mortality was the highest in Bengal after the Central Provinces, Orissa, and Burma.[15]

Different officials who wrote articles and began to collate the fragmentary data from hospital returns presented a picture of the extent of puerperal sepsis and stated anaemia and eclampsia to be the leading causes of maternal mortality.[16] In 1936, the Indian Research Fund Association (IRFA)—an organization set up in 1911 with the aim of recruiting and training medical researchers and for channelling funds (government and private) to approved medical research programmes—provided a grant of Rs 7,500 for two women doctors to support a statistical inquiry into maternal mortality in Calcutta.[17] The results of the investigation of 595 deaths during June–December 1936 revealed that 505 deaths were due to maternal causes. Childbearing alone was responsible for 80.4 per cent of deaths (from sepsis, anaemia, and toxaemias).[18] By 1938, it seemed that 'child-bearing exacts a toll of lives in India at least four or five times greater than in those countries where serious attention has been given to the protection of motherhood'.[19]

If we look at a more nuanced picture, it can be seen from evidence provided by the Royal Commission of Labour in India (1928) and Report of the Age of Consent Committee (1928–9), that in tea plantations,

Asansol mines, and mill areas, infant death rate during 1919–29 was lower than the provincial decennial average. Birth rate in tea gardens was higher than in rural areas.[20] It seems that despite poverty and exploitation, because of the less strenuous nature of work than in mines and mills, and some amount of financial support provided by planters, conditions in tea gardens, rather than in rural towns, were more congenial to childbirth and survival of the infant. British doctors, however, pointed out that untrained and dirty midwifery accounted for a large number of deaths in plantations. In fact, as pointed out in an earlier chapter, most Western observers blamed Indian social customs, rituals, and dirty midwifery for high maternal and infant death rates in Bengal.[21] British officials claimed that the practices of traditional Indian midwives and unhygienic environment were mainly responsible for the unusually high rate of infant mortality in Bengal.[22]

Mary Frances Billington had written earlier:

> That infant mortality is very high is not on account of evil intent, but is due to the appalling ignorance of the *dhais*, the professional class of midwives or monthly nurses, whose methods of treatment are simply barbarous and, indeed if viewed in the light of our Western scientific knowledge, seem as if it would be enough to kill every unfortunate victim upon whom they were practised.[23]

This trend continued even in the 1920s. It was noted in the Bengal Census of 1921:

> Much has been said and written of the evils of early marriage, resulting in the survival of child-widows condemned to a life of austerity and very often of drudgery and so on, but to the critic of these statistics the evil which does far more harm to other women of this country is the custom that ordains, that a married woman must not only be married but live the life of a married woman immediately she attains puberty.[24]

Thus British critics focused on the prevalent practices of child marriage and consummation immediately after puberty as other reasons behind high maternal and infant mortality in Bengal. In 1909, Major W.W. Clemensha, sanitary commissioner of Bengal, pointed out: 'Out of 2700 children that die within the first month (in Calcutta), more than 1200 or nearly 50% come under the hands of premature birth and debility at birth.... Probably early marriage is the preponderating factor.'[25]

From the 1920s onwards, Indian social customs and sexual practices also became objects of international—apart from colonial—scrutiny. The New York journalist Katherine Mayo, who visited India in 1925, in her book *Mother India* (1927) launched a devastating attack on Indian social customs.[26] She presented quite a provocative description of sexual perversions and of the inequalities of the patriarchal system in Indian society to convey the message that India lacked political maturity. Mayo's account, in fact, used the bare facts of population growth, infant mortality, and death rates to justify British rule over India. Moreover, the book continued the British–Indian tradition of singling out Bengal for moral condemnation.[27]

In the face of accumulating pressure, the Indian government decided to set up a commission to investigate the state of affairs in the country, and in June 1928, the Age of Consent Committee was established under the chairmanship of M.V. Joshi, who had served as home member of the executive council of the governor of the Central Provinces.[28] India had already passed the Act XXIX of 1925, which had raised the age of consent to thirteen in marital and fourteen in non-marital cases. But apparently, very few were aware of the Act.

The Joshi Committee's terms of reference included investigation of all questions/issues surrounding the age of consent and to examine the effects of the 1925 Act. It was composed of ten Indians and one British woman doctor. In the summer of 1928, they formulated a questionnaire and sent it directly to 6,000 selected people or public bodies and to a further 1,930 persons through local governments.[29] Among other things, questions were asked to probe the effects of early intercourse on girls and their future progeny, and women's attitudes to the custom and the existing legislation. According to the committee, 'the primary object of promoting legislation fixing the age of Marriage or raising the age of Consent in marital cases is to minimize the risks of maternal and infantile mortality and to increase the chances of a longer and healthier life of the citizens.'[30] The Committee compiled nine volumes of evidence, containing both oral and written statements from witnesses all over the country. The Age of Consent Committee emphasized the fact that the low birth rate in Bengal was caused by early sexual intercourse and the subsequent emaciation of women.[31] British observers, however, admitted that poverty—particularly among the labouring classes—contributed to maternal death.

One way of addressing the problem of maternal mortality and poor health was to organize and devise means of making individuals, particularly mothers, aware of health issues. The Association for the Provision of Health Visitors and Maternity Supervisors was started in 1918 with Henry Sharp (the secretary of the education department of the government of India) as chairman and Dr M.I. Balfour as honorary secretary. In the following year was established the Lady Chelmsford All India League for Maternity and Child Welfare, which coordinated the maternal and child benefit works in all the provinces of British India. With its headquarters at the Viceregal Lodge in Simla, it was intended to act as a central agency for collecting information regarding child welfare and to impart training to lady health visitors. In July 1923, the public health commissioner of the government of India sent out the programme for a National Health Week, as formulated by Professor Bostock Hill in England, with a suggestion that such a programme be adopted in India. In October 1923, the National Health Week was observed in England.[32]

Organization of baby shows and welfare exhibitions, and distribution of prizes and rewards for childcare became part of the programmes arranged by Dufferin hospitals. Public health education, child welfare centres, and baby shows were patterned on the Western model, which would supposedly provide better health and longer lifespan for women and children. The Baby Week movement was inaugurated in 1924 throughout Bengal as part of an all-India movement. The Indian Red Cross Society Welfare Division, opened by Lady Lytton in January, took part in it. Lectures and exhibitions were organized in different districts to celebrate baby weeks. This gradually became an annual feature.

One of the most important activities of the Lady Chelmsford All India League for Maternity and Child Welfare was the publication of literature for sale on maternity and child welfare subjects. It was the only organization involved in this kind of publication. Another important work of the League was supporting health schools in different provinces. The Bengal school for welfare workers was started in 1924 and eight students were trained in the inaugural year. The Countess of Lytton, as the president of the League, in her address on the occasion of the inauguration of the school and a hostel put emphasis on the importance of the selection and training of suitable people to become health visitors 'as the establishment of Welfare centres was in its infancy and pioneers had to be especially capable'. Of the eight students who successfully completed their training in the first year, '2 students of the English course will have charge of Welfare Centres being opened up in Jute mills, one has charge of a Calcutta Indian Baby clinic. Of the students of the vernacular course, three have charge of Calcutta Indian Baby Clinic one has returned to Dacca'. The school budget was met entirely through voluntary contributions and it was regretted that the local government did not come forward to give financial help.[33]

Internationally, the post–World War I period (also) witnessed a lot of concern for the health of the labouring women. The debate on maternity benefit and maternity leave was initiated by the Convention of the Washington International Labour Conference, which met in October 1919. It was suggested that six weeks' leave before and after childbirth, along with sufficient benefits, should be granted to women in commercial and industrial undertakings. In Bengal, women in tea plantations received benefits from the planters on a voluntary basis. Piecemeal benefit schemes were set up in the early 1920s by the management of the Baranagore and Kelvin Jute Mills.[34] The maternity and child welfare centre at the Titagar Mills, started in March 1923, offered the service of a qualified health supervisor, and introduced classes for indigenous midwives, instruction classes for expectant mothers, baby clinics, and sewing classes to teach mothers to tailor baby cloths. The centre provided soaps for babies, but no food for mothers or milk for babies. During the 1920s this model scheme was imitated in many mills. Women were asked to learn hygiene and modesty before they would gain the right of maintenance during maternity.[35] In the early 1920s, the Asansol Mines Board of Health employed three trained midwives. By 1929, training classes for indigenous midwives were also opened and the latter were given fully equipped midwifery bags.[36]

Local Efforts

In 1919, the Government of Bengal appointed a Child Welfare Committee consisting of medical personnel to give advice on measures to be adopted in order to promote child welfare and reduce infant mortality.[37] The report of the Committee, submitted in 1921, recommended, among other measures, education of dhais or untrained midwives. Local bodies such as district boards and municipalities, which were primarily responsible for maternal and infant welfare, appointed lady doctors attached with dispensaries and hospitals. The local authorities received annual government grants of Rs 15,000 for imparting training to pupil nurses and dhais in state and private hospitals.

The year 1921 saw the inauguration of the scheme to train indigenous village dhais, and a number of district boards established training centres for this purpose. The department of public health did not exercise any direct supervision over the training of dhais or over any of the maternal and child welfare clinics. The school hygiene branch of the Bengal sanitary department inaugurated in September 1920 (consisting of one deputy sanitary commissioner who was designated assistant director of public health from 1921, one medical inspector, and one medical inspectress of schools), organized dhai-training classes and assisted at the annual baby week and health exhibitions.

The public health department sanctioned grants-in-aid for different voluntary organizations like the Bengal Health Welfare Committee of the Provincial Branch of the Indian Red Cross Society and Saroj Nalini Dutt Memorial Association.[38] The latter worked for maternal and child-care and for exhibitions and propaganda.[39] Small grants from provincial revenues were given towards the maintenance of a few maternity and child welfare centres such as Barisal maternity clinic, Rangpur maternity clinic, Dacca Maternity Trust, Orakandi and Chapra and Chittagong hill tracts maternity clinics, Kalia maternity and child welfare centre, and the Servants of Human Society.[40] A certain number of maternity beds or wards were provided in large maternity hospitals. Calcutta possessed special women's hospitals, maintained by the Bengal government and the Dufferin Fund; two more (Chittaranjan Seva Sadan, and Ramakrishna Sishu Mangal and Matri Pratisthan) were maintained using local funds.[41]

In the 1920s, the health publicity and propaganda branch of the public health department of Bengal gradually expanded to carry out extensive works including organization of magic-lantern shows, film shows, and so forth. By 1928, films were regarded as the best propaganda instrument. The ward health associations of the Calcutta Corporation arranged lantern lectures and exhibitions to educate mothers about health care for themselves as well as children. Health films—dealing, among other subjects, with maternity and child welfare—were produced and shown by the Bengal public health department.[42]

The government also extended financial assistance in the form of capital grants, to the extent of 50 per cent of the total expenses, to local bodies and recognized voluntary organizations for the establishment and maintenance of welfare centres.[43] Each centre, serving a population of 10,000, was under the management of a local committee (40 per cent of each committee was composed of official members such as district magistrates, district judges and 60 per cent were other members, of whom 30 per cent were women representatives). The staff of each welfare centre consisted of a health visitor who was responsible for the conduct of the welfare services. Her work was supervised by the lady superintendent of maternity and child welfare, appointed in September 1939. The superintendent was entrusted with the responsibility of promoting and coordinating the necessary activities, educating public opinion, investigating probable reasons for maternal and infant mortality, and suggesting means for improvement.[44] From February 1944, a government-sanctioned scheme was started for free distribution of milk and clothes to needy and poor mothers.[45]

In December 1932, the All India Institute of Hygiene and Public Health (AIIHPH) was formally opened in Calcutta. The funding for the maternity and child welfare section of this institute was provided by the Dufferin Fund and Red Cross Association of India (RCAI).[46] Dr Jean Orkney of the WMS took charge of its work. Two students completed the diploma course in maternity and child welfare in 1934, which was started by the Calcutta School of Tropical Medicine and Hygiene in 1933, followed by two more students in 1935. But in 1935–6 there were no takers for the diploma course at all, and only one each for the years 1936–7, 1937–8, and 1938–9. Six students successfully completed the diploma course in 1939–40 and 1940–1.[47]

A clinic was set up to serve in Ward 8 of the Calcutta Corporation. Within a year, the maternity and child welfare programme was said to be reaching more than half the pregnant women in the ward and providing effective antenatal and postnatal services. By 1938, attendance at the clinic had reached 8,456. Moreover, there were 7,500 home visits by the two health visitors and 202 antenatal visits were made by the midwives.[48] A parallel scheme was launched at the Clive Jute Mill in Calcutta to introduce diploma students to 'the problems of women in industry, maternity benefits, administration of crèches and the general social-welfare scheme required under industrial conditions.'[49]

The manner in which responsibility for the maternity and child welfare section of the AIIHPH and the Maternity and Welfare Clinic—which it subsequently established—was passed to the Red Cross, the Dufferin Fund, the Marwari community, the Calcutta Football Association and Turf Club, and others[50] proved that provisions for maternal and child health care continued to be of relatively low priority in official schemes. Responsibility for maternal and child health in general was still relegated to the voluntary sector. Following the example of philanthropic organizations, like the Dufferin Fund, in 1903 Lady Curzon created the Victoria Memorial Scholarship Scheme for training midwives.[51]

Nationalism, Women's Organizations, and Health Reforms

The work of the wives of Viceroys in the sphere of maternal and childcare—when coupled with racial arrogance—often served to provoke nationalist resentment. Events like baby shows were condemned as being an insult to Indian motherhood by a section of the nationalist Bengali press.[52] In the period following World War I, nationalist politics encouraged Indian women activists to organize baby shows and work for improvement in the conditions of childbirth. As has been argued by Judy Whitehead, by the 1920s, the colonized middle classes sought 'to project themselves as the legitimate heirs of "the nation" pitted against a colonial bureaucracy increasingly wary of alienating its narrowing base of political support.'[53] The predominant concern in the nationalist circle was with proper development of children, who were considered the future of the nation. In Indian nationalism, the health of the nation was increasingly linked to the goal of Swaraj. In the early twentieth century, the social work organized by educated middle-class women who formed *mahila samitis* (women's associations) was motivated by nationalist politics. The public health models of motherhood adopted by reformers and women's organizations in this period focused on the need to promote better hygienic practices in homes through social service. A major part of the responsibility for improving the health of the nation fell on self-sacrificing mothers.

The Sarda Act of 1929 (like the Act of 1891) saw the convergence of medical opinion and nationalist agitation over raising the age of permissible sexual intercourse in marriage from twelve to fourteen. Doctors spoke out publicly in favour of raising the age of consent and against the practice of child marriage, calling it 'barbarous'.[54] The mild reaction to the Sarda Act of 1929 that prohibited early marriages stands in contrast to the controversies aroused by the ban on sati, the law permitting widow remarriage, and the Age of Consent Act of 1891. Judy Whitehead argues convincingly that this shift in nationalist opinion reflects the entry of women's nationalist organizations into the political sphere, the changing balance of class relations in late colonial India, and the increasing prestige of biomedical sciences in legal debates.[55] Indian observers often blamed insanitary housing conditions, insufficient supply of milk, as well as scarcity and high price of cow's milk (apart from bad midwifery and the social custom of early marriage) for high rates of infant mortality. Inadequate and insufficient maternal diet was one of the major causes of racial decay. The Bengali witnesses before the Age of Consent Committee, including women doctors and health workers, pointed out that the low birth rate accompanied by high infant mortality was due to malnutrition of overworked women and the economic decline of the province.[56] In addition, they argued, it was not the mother's age at birth which exhausted women, but the high frequency of births. The nationalist press criticized the government for the supply of poor-quality milk to places like the Calcutta Medical College Hospital and also for their negligence of problems like food adulteration and bad housing conditions.[57] New knowledge of nutrition was harnessed to strengthen efforts to improve maternal and infant health. Feeding the wrong foods to infants was also blamed for poor child health. Research articles published in the *Journal of Association of Medical Women in India* (*JAMWI*) also revealed the high degree of malnutrition and sickness among mothers and infants.[58]

Meredith Borthwick has narrated how, since the late nineteenth century, educated women who had mastered midwifery tried to put their new knowledge to use by helping others. Sailabala Sen, whose mother was a midwife, learnt midwifery from a doctor and served her family members, neighbours, as well as the poor and the needy. She had mastered the skill so well from books that she could attend difficult deliveries successfully.[59] Nalinibala Chaudhuri, mentioned earlier (in Chapter 3), set up a training centre for midwives in Sylhet.[60]

Associations formed by middle-class women organized social work, including child and maternal welfare, first at an all-India level and then in different parts of Bengal.[61] At the all-India level, the Women's Indian Association (WIA) was formed in 1917 in Madras by Margaret Cousins, an Irish feminist, theosophist, and musician,[62] and Dorothy Jinarajadasa, also an Irish feminist. Membership was open to both Indians and Europeans. Between 1917 and 1922, the WIA, through articles in *Stri Dharma*, stressed the necessity of educating girls in child welfare, first aid, hygiene, biology, and the sciences, apart from other subjects, to make them aware of their future duties to the nation as caretakers of healthy, strong children. Women doctors like Mary Scharlieb[63] and Muthulakshmi Reddi[64] supported training women in domestic or personal hygiene, sanitation, and child and maternity welfare.

The WIA also put forward the argument that women's education and right to vote would result in medical benefits to their children and for the nation as a whole.[65] Others also used this line of argument. In 1913, Saroj Nalini Dutt, wife of Gurusaday Dutt and a prominent reformer, founded a mahila samiti in Patna and used arguments based on public health to defend the claim for the extension of women's education thus:

> If you think that women know all they need to know without education, then how would you account for the appalling rate of infant mortality in India?...Education in the laws of health and hygiene alone can lift this curse of ignorance from the mothers.... Mahila samitis will bring the knowledge of the sciences to the very doors of women.[66]

Saroj Nalini created mahila samitis in many areas including Pabna, Birbhum, and Bankura. One important aim was to train women in domestic science and hygiene. In 1925, Gurusaday Dutt founded the SNDMA, an umbrella organization for mahila samitis and village or municipal women's groups. By 1929, there were about 250 autonomous groups all over Bengal, and it rose to 305 by 1930.

Classes on hygiene were arranged and baby shows were also organized. In 1925, the mahila samiti of Bankura celebrated a baby week. Latika Basu, the secretary of the Chittaranjan Seva Sadan, a special women's hospital founded in 1926, informed the Age of Consent Committee about its purpose of training nurses and midwives for village work.[67] Calcutta nationalist celebrities such as Jyotirmoyi Ganguli and Latika Ghose were among the founding members of the SNDMA. Many groups were founded by local women in villages or urban neighbourhoods, which tried to attract lower-middle-class membership. They conducted training programmes and stressed individual participation that aimed at female literacy, reviving village crafts, teaching needle work, and so on. Female cooperation was regarded essential for village reconstruction, and improving traditional midwifery and conditions in the lying-in room were priorities of the members.[68] Some of the early members at district or village levels excelled at midwifery.

Sometimes a mahila samiti would set up maternity clinics or install clean maternity wards in local hospitals. These were managed by only women and helped to liberate mothers from the depressing conditions in traditional anturghars. Classes on maintaining hygiene during birth were also arranged for traditional midwives. By 1929, there were over 250 samitis all over Bengal and almost all had worked towards improving the conditions of birth and worked towards the organization of baby shows. In 1929, in Kidderpur, near the Calcutta docks, a lying-in room was opened where local female factory workers could come for their deliveries free of charge.[69]

Birth Control

Rai Sahib Harbilas Sarda, a prominent Arya Samajist who was also deputy leader of the Nationalist Party, introduced a bill in February 1927 to prevent the marriages of girls below the age of twelve and boys below fourteen.[70] The Child Marriage Restraint Act of 1929 (popularly known as the Sarda Act, after Rai Sahib Harbilas Sarda), as noted earlier, raised the minimum age of marriage for girls from ten to twelve years.[71] The WIA organized a house to house campaign to collect signatures in support of Sarda's bill in 1927. On 8 September 1928, in Bengal, a large number of women gathered at Albert Hall to demand that the age of marriage be raised to sixteen for women and eighteen or twenty for men. The SNDMA supported the bill and even tried to implement the reform in the villages. Geraldine Forbes has observed that in dealing with the Sarda Act Indian women for the first time made 'their presence felt as a pressure group to be reckoned with in matters of social legislation'.[72] In its final report, the Sarda Committee suggested the use of contraceptives as one of the alternatives for achieving the objective of the proposed law. In fact, already in the early 1920s, Indian men had started discussions on the need for birth control and made efforts to establish institutions to provide information on contraception. Foreigners like Margaret Sanger also entered the debate. In 1931, the census figures first demonstrated a substantial demographic increase of 10.6 per cent.[73] J.H. Hutton, the census commissioner in 1931, pointed out that what was needed in India, instead of the 'luxury' of baby weeks, were precautions to reduce the birth rate.[74]

At the sixth session of the All India Women's Conference (AIWC) in Madras in December 1931, Rani Lakshmi Rajwade, who had received her medical education in Bombay and Great Britain, proposed the following resolution:

> In view of the immense increase in the population of the country and having regard to the poverty and the low physical standard of the people, this Conference is in favour of appointing a committee of medical women to study and recommend ways and means of educating the public to regulate the size of their families.[75]

Rajwade's resolution was supported—among others—by Renuka Ray, a volunteer social worker from Calcutta. Ray argued that Indian women 'should tear the veil of false modesty and prejudice if they wanted the race to be full of vigour, health and happiness'.[76] Rajwade's resolution was opposed by women like Khadijah Begum Ferozuddin, a Muslim professor at the Government College for Women in Lahore and Miss Ouwerkerk, a Dutch Christian missionary teacher in Trivandrum. Muthulakshmi Reddi supported the Gandhian ideal of self-control. After the defeat of Rajawade's proposal, Reddi secured the passage of a resolution calling for education in mothercraft and fathercraft.

In Calcutta, in early 1935, Colonel Owen Berkeley-Hill, a retired member of the Indian Medical Service, formed the Women's Welfare Society with a group of associates. They started a birth control clinic in June 1935 at Dufferin Hospital, but the Hospital would not allow the clinic to advertise, and so it attracted few clients. By September 1936, the Women's Welfare Society decided to operate an independent clinic in rented facilities under the direction of Dr Margaret Neal, and to broaden its scope to include contraception, child guidance, vocational guidance, and sex hygiene. This action was reflected in a change of its name to the Marriage Welfare and Child Guidance Association. The independent clinic of this Association, which did not accept women with incomes over Rs 200, was active until 1942, when it closed as the Japanese invasion of Burma threatened Calcutta.

The subject of birth control became a controversial matter. It was debated not only among members of the AIWC but among male as well as female physicians. Although some women physicians were eager to embrace birth control as an additional knowledge necessary to further their professional careers, there were others who regarded contraceptives as potentially dangerous to the socio-moral fabric of society.

The debate among women physicians about the legitimacy of birth control occurred largely within the *JAMWI*.[77] Mrs Lilias M. Jeffries's article named 'Prevention', published in May 1921, was the first one on the subject of birth control published in the journal.[78] In her conclusion, Jeffries emphasized how birth control would ensure eugenic results, improve the race, and eliminate the 'unfit'. Dr Ruth Young, director of the Maternity and Child Welfare Bureau, in her essay titled 'Medical Women and Conception Control', published in *JAMWI* in 1934, argued that medical women should acquaint themselves with the subject of birth control.[79] Margaret Balfour, an important and well-known woman physician who worked mainly in Punjab from 1892 to 1924, wanted that the knowledge of birth control should be under the control of trained physicians only. Thus, she was anxious to establish biomedical hegemony over the emerging field of contraceptives within the domain of women's health care. There were a few Indian women doctors in the Association of Medical Women in India, some of whom contributed to the ongoing discussions on birth control in the *JAMWI*. Dr Miss Jerbanoo Mistry was one such doctor who lent her support to birth control.[80]

Despite Gandhi's opposition to birth control, the AIWC passed a resolution on the issue in 1932 at its Lucknow session. It was stated:

> This conference feels that on account of low physique of women, high infant mortality, and increasing poverty of the country, married men and women should be instructed in methods of birth control in recognized clinics. It calls upon all municipalities and local bodies to open such centers and invites the special help of the medical authorities towards the resolution of this important problem.[81]

In the 1936 AIWC session, the resolution on birth control was carried through with eighty-three voting for and twenty-five against it. At the Nagpur session of the AIWC in 1937, the resolution was passed with only one dissenting vote.

In the face of Gandhian opposition to the use of mechanical and chemical contraceptives, Indian women supporters of birth control acted very cautiously. Women like Laxmibai Rajwade, Lakhmi Menon, Begum Hamid Ali, Kamaladevi Chattopadhyaya, and Margaret Cousins were strong advocates of contraceptive usage. They expressed their commitment to women's traditional role as mothers and used the health script to blunt any potentially radical nature of their opinion. Defending the demand for birth control, Laxmibai Rajwade argued 'that child and maternal mortality are directly related to frequent child birth. The mothers grow anaemic, emaciated, are easy victims to disease while the offspring of such mothers are none better'.[82]

It has been pointed out by some scholars that on the specific issue of birth control, Indian feminists were caught between a contradictory impulse of simultaneously representing Indian women as repositories of national traditions as well as embodiments of modernity in an emerging nation.[83] Undoubtedly, feminist politics was neither static nor homogenous, nor did it articulate the issue of birth control from a singular unified perspective.

Kamaladevi Chattopadhyaya, the first organizing secretary of the AIWC and a member of the Socialist wing of the Indian National Congress, argued that 'from the point of view of national benefit birth control is necessary for reasons of health, social and economic considerations'.[84] These middle-class female advocates, no doubt, selectively deployed the dominant discourses of Malthusianism, eugenics, and nationalism to make a public case for supporting birth control.

They, however, mainly represented the interests of middle-class, Hindu, upper-caste, or Muslim *ashraf* (high-born) women. It has been rightly pointed out that 'it was the privileged and elite articulations of middle-class Indian women (even though these were internally fractured) that became part of the public debates on birth control, which did not allow much room for subaltern concerns or agendas to shape and determine these debates in the twentieth century'.[85]

***

In late colonial Bengal, health education aiming at maternal and child welfare became a site for interaction between state agencies promoting sanitation and public health, and Indian politicians and social reformers endorsing public health as central to nation-building. It can be argued that events like baby shows indicate the desire of both British officials and Indian political leaders to move from private to public spaces and relationships. Their role was basically educative but they were designed to create clients for maternal and child welfare centres and to open doors for lady health visitors.

It has been pointed out that 'professional health visitors represented the movement of Western medical care and the state into Indian homes'; maternal and child welfare centres, often collaborators of local governments and private philanthropists, were to be permanent sites for primarily preventive and only secondarily curative work for infants and for the education of their mothers, primarily of lower social and economic classes.[86]

In late colonial India, works carried out by professional health visitors undoubtedly represented the movement of Western medical care and the state into Indian homes. Propaganda efforts of maternal and child welfare centres, works of school inspectors, and other such moves aiming at health education also meant that the health system was turning from repressive approaches to constructive approaches aiming at garnering the participation of clients. Preventive health care aimed at the health education of individuals, which became the public health model in the early twentieth century, is traditionally conceived as an asset within health care because it provides information and suggests alternatives to individuals, families, or groups to prevent disease and promote health. From this perspective, health education seems to be a healthy practice and a weapon for empowering patients.

Yet, sometimes health education practices involved the imposition of 'truths' about health, in which the patient lost control of her or his own body. Instead of choice, the patient experienced the governing of her or his body or family from outside. The concept of biopower provides a critique of health education, which actually seemed to become part of surveillance medicine and contributed to the management of social and individual bodies.[87]

It may further be pointed out in the context of colonial India that the hygienic model naturalized the role of women as biological reproducers. Moreover, maternal and child health care through promotion of health education were part of a shift to preventive care, which did not address the problem of poverty. This was problematic in that it aimed to provide health education for poor women and babies who needed structural changes in the economy in order to survive and mature as healthy individuals.

From another point of view, as argued elsewhere,[88] the benefits derived from efforts at improving hygienic knowledge or domestic health behaviour in case of the general population in British Bengal was not very noteworthy. It seems that the campaign for adopting better individual health practices could bring about dramatic health improvements only when it was pre-existed by a macro-sanitary and administrative infrastructure, better nutritional status, and moreover, when applied to a relatively well-fed and well-housed population, like the Indian army.[89] The propaganda for birth control through adoption of contraceptive means also did not really lead to any noticeable improvement of reproductive health. The maternal death rate in Bengal showed an upward trend between 1929 and 1938, rising from around 7 per cent to nearly 11 per cent. Between 1939 and 1944, it fluctuated between nearly 9 per cent and more than 10 per cent. The infant death rate also presented a dismal picture, fluctuating between nearly 150 and more than 200 per 1,000 during the same period.[90]

Notes and References

1. Antoinette Burton, *Dwelling in the Archive: Women Writing House, Home, and History in Late Colonial India* (New York: Oxford University Press, 2003), p. 9. Cited in Sanjam Ahluwalia, *Reproductive Restraints: Birth Control in India 1877–1947* (New Delhi: Permanent Black, 2008), p. 42.

2. Partha Chatterjee, 'The Nationalist Resolution of the Woman's Question', in *Recasting Women: Essays in Colonial History*, edited by Kumkum Sangari and Sudesh Vaid (New Delhi: Kali for Women, 1989), pp. 233–54.

3. For discussions on nineteenth-century debates on masculinity and nationalism, see Uma Chakravarty, 'Whatever Happened to the Vedic Dasi?' in Sangari and Vaid, *Recasting Women*, pp. 27–87; Mrinalini Sinha, *Colonial Masculinity: The 'Manly Englishman' and the 'Effeminate Bengali' in the Late Nineteenth Century* (Manchester: Manchester University Press, 1995); John Rosselli, 'The Self-Image of Effeteness: Physical Education and Nationalism in Nineteenth-Century Bengal', *Past and Present* 87 (February 1980): 121–48.

4. Barbara Ramusack, 'Embattled Advocates: The Debate over Birth Control in India, 1920–1940', *Journal of Women's History* 1, no. 2 (1989): 34–64; S. Anandhi, 'Reproductive Bodies and Regulated Sexuality: Birth Control Debates in Early Twentieth-Century Tamil Nadu', in *A Question of Silence? The Sexual Economies of Modern India*, edited by Mary John and Janaki Nair (New Delhi: Kali for Women 1998), pp. 139–66; Mausumi Manna, 'Approach towards Birth Control: Indian Women in the Early Twentieth Century', *IESHR* 35, no. 1 (1998): 35–51; Sarah Hodges, *Conjugality, Progeny and Progress: Family and Modernity in India* (PhD diss., University of Chicago, 1999), pp. 160–208; Sanjam Ahluwalia, *Reproductive Restraints Birth Control in India 1877–1947* (New Delhi: Permanent Black, 2008).

5. See Sujata Mukherjee, 'Disciplining the Body? Health Care for Women and Children in Early Twentieth-Century Bengal', in *Disease and Medicine in India: A Historical Overview*, edited by Deepak Kumar (New Delhi: Tulika Books, 2001), pp. 198–214.

6. F.B. Smith, *The People's Health, 1830–1910* (London: Croom Helm, 1979), p. 114. Cited in Sumit Guha, *Health and Population in South Asia From Earliest Times to the Present* (New Delhi: Permanent Black, 2001), p. 133.

7. Anna Davin, 'Imperialism and Motherhood', *History Workshop Journal* 5 (1978): 43.

8. See Judy Whitehead, 'Modernising the Motherhood Archetype: Public Health Models and the Child Marriage Restraint Act of 1929', in *Social Reform, Sexuality and the State*, edited by Patricia Uberoi (New Delhi: SAGE Publications, 1996), pp. 188–209.

9. Mukherjee, 'Disciplining the Body?'

10. David Arnold, 'Official Attitudes to Population, Birth Control and Reproductive Health in India, 1921–1946', in *Reproductive Health in India: History, Politics, Controversies,* edited by Sarah Hodges (New Delhi: Orient Longman, 2006), pp. 22–50, 37.

11. The WMS was established by the Government of India in 1914. The number of its members was small—with only forty women doctors in active service in the mid-1930s—compared to the Indian Medical Service, which was nearly a thousand strong, and its responsibilities were largely confined to the treatment of women and children, and the staffing of women's hospitals. Moreover, it formed only about a tenth of all qualified medical women practising in India in the 1930s. Unlike journals like the *IMG* (started from the 1860s) and the *Indian Journal of Medical Research* (first appeared in 1913), the *Journal of the Association of Medical Women in India* published a large number of articles and essays written by WMS doctors on obstetrics, gynaecology, and women's health in general.

12. D. Curjel, *Improvement of the Conditions of Childbirth in India.* Calcutta: Bengal Secretariat Book Depot, 1918.

13. *Report of the Municipal Administration of Calcutta,* 1920–1, pp. 67–8, available at National Library, Kolkata.

14. *Census of India, 1921,* vol. 1, pp. 209, 230. Cited in Mukherjee, 'Disciplining the Body?', p. 202n26.

15. Resolution no. 1176 P.H., dated 23 July 1940, of the Government of Bengal, Department of Public Health and Local Self Government, on the Bengal Public health Report, 1938. Cited in Mukherjee, 'Disciplining the Body?', p. 202n27.

16. Margaret Balfour, 'Maternal Mortality in Childbirth in India', *JAMWI* 16, no. 1 (1928): 5–25.

17. See Arnold, 'Official Attitudes to Population', p. 43.

18. Arnold, 'Official Attitudes to Population', p. 43.

19. Central Advisory Board of Health (CABH), *Report on Maternity and Child Welfare Work in India by Special Committee (1938)* (Simla: Manager, Government of India Press, 1939), p. 24.

20. Dagmar Engels, *Beyond Purdah? Women in Bengal 1890–1939* (New Delhi: Oxford University Press, 1996), p. 151.

21. See Chapter 3 of this volume.

22. *Census of India,* 1911, vol. 4, part I, p. 30. Cited in Mukherjee, 'Disciplining the Body?', pp. 203–4.

23. Mary Frances Billington, *Women in India* (New Delhi: Sri Satguru Publications, 1987 [1895]), p. 2. Also cited in Malavika Karlekar, *Voices from*

Within: Early Personal Narratives of Bengali Women (New Delhi: Oxford University Press, 1991), p. 53.

24. *Census of India*, 1921, vol. 5, part I, p. 255. Also cited in Engels, *Beyond Purdah? Women in Bengal*, p. 130n36.

25. *Census of India*, 1911, vol. 4, part I, p. 31.

26. Geraldine Forbes, 'Women and Modernity: The Issue of Child Marriage in India', *Women's Studies International Quarterly* 2 (1979): 412. Also cited in Engels, *Beyond Purdah? Women in Bengal*, p. 145n103.

27. Katherine Mayo, *Mother India* (London: Jonathan Cape Ltd, 1927), p. 118.

28. Government of India, Home/Judicial, 382/1927, notes, pp. 9–10.

29. For details, see Barbara N. Ramusack, 'Women's Organizations and Social Change: The Age-of-marriage Issue in India', in *Women and World Change: Equity Issues in Development*, edited by Naomi Black and Ann Baker Cottrell (Beverly Hills, California: SAGE Publications, 1981), pp. 198–216; Geraldine Forbes, *The New Cambridge History of India*, vol. 4, part 2, *Women in Modern India* (Cambridge: Cambridge University Press, 1998), pp. 87–90; Whitehead, 'Modernizing the Motherhood Archetype'; Mrinalini Sinha, 'Lineage of the "Indian" Modern: Rhetoric, Agency and the Sarda Act in Late Colonial India', in *Gender, Sexuality and Colonial Modernity*, edited by Antoinette Burton (London: Routledge, 2000), pp. 207–21.

30. *Age of Consent Report, 76*, *Census of India*, 1911, vol. 5, part I, p. 269.

31. In July 1923, the public health commissioner of the Government of India sent out the programme for a National Health Week, as formulated by Professor Bostock Hill in England, with a suggestion that such a programme be adopted in India. In October 1923, the National Health Week was observed in England. See Mukherjee, 'Disciplining the Body?', pp. 205–6.

32. *Annual Report of the National Association for Supplying Medical Aid by Women to Women in India*, 1925. Also cited in Mukherjee, 'Disciplining the Body?', pp. 205–6.

33. For discussions on maternity benefits for women labourers in jute mills in Bengal, see Engels, *Beyond Purdah? Women in Bengal*; Samita Sen, *Women and Labour in Late Colonial India: The Bengal Jute Industry* (Cambridge: Cambridge University Press, 1999).

34. WBSA, Comm./Comm., December 1924, A48, and July 1925, A47, p. 68 and July 1927, A6-8, 6–7; 'Curjel Report', Appendix A, pp. xiv–xxv.

35. 'Curjel Report', Appendix A, pp. xvii–xviii, Appendix E, 7; RCLI, v, 1, pp. 32, 35, 181.

36. The Child Welfare Committee was appointed by Resolution no. 72T-San., of the GB. Local Self Government (LSG) Department, dated 28 May 1919.

The Committee was made permanent by Resolution no. 1122 Public Health dated 8 April 1921.

37. Letter from A.D. Stewart, DPH (offg), to the Secy, to the GB, Calcutta, 30 June 1925, LSG Dept, F. No. Public Health 2-S-2, progs A2–3, August 1926.

38. *Bengal Public Health Report*, 1936, p. 96.

39. *Bengal Public Health Report*, 1938, p. 111.

40. *Bengal Public Health Report*, 1936, p. 100.

41. *Bengal Public Health Report*, 1938, p. 111.

42. *Bengal Public Health Report*, 1927, p. 70. Also cited in 'Disciplining the Body?', p. 207.

43. See Kabita Ray, *History of Public Health: Colonial Bengal 1921–1947* (Calcutta: K.P. Bagchi & Company, 1998), p. 315.

44. *Bengal Public Health Report*, 1940, pp. 115–16.

45. *Bengal Public Health Report*, 1944, p. 22.

46. Arnold, 'Official Attitudes to Population', p. 41.

47. *Summary Report of the Work Done in the All India Institute of Hygiene and Public Health for the Period 1940 to 1944* (Calcutta: 1945).

48. *Annual Report of the All India Institute of Hygiene and Public Health* (Calcutta: 1938), p. 45.

49. *Annual Report*, All India Institute of Hygiene and Public Health, 1935, 41–2. The most detailed account of the clinic's work is to be found in the *Annual Report of the All India Institute of Hygiene and Public Health* (Calcutta: 1937), pp. 46–57.

50. Annual Report, All India Institute of Hygiene and Public Health (Calcutta: 1934), pp. 12–13, 23.

51. In the absence of follow-up supervision, village midwives returned to old habits after attending a few classes. Margaret I. Balfour and Ruth Young, *The Work of Medical Women in India* (London: Oxford University Press, 1929), pp. 130–2.

52. Such sentiments were fuelled by, for example, the attitudes of women like the Vicereine Lady Reading, who founded the 'Lady Reading All-India Hospital Fund' to raise money for the 'Lady Reading Hospital for Indian Women and Children' in Shimla, visited a zenana hospital, a child welfare centre, a health school, a nurses' home, and a fund-raising occasion every second day during her 1921 Christmas stay in Calcutta. She perceived these visits almost as outings to the zoo. IOLR, MSS.Eur.E 316.10, Lady Reading Papers, Schedule for the Calcutta Visit, 3 to 22 December 1921. See Engels, *Beyond Purdah? Women in Bengal*, p. 147.

53. See Whitehead, 'Modernising the Motherhood Archetype', p. 187.

54. David Arnold, *Colonizing the Body: State Medicine and Epidemic Disease in Nineteenth-Century India* (Berkeley, California: University of California Press, 1993), p. 265.

55. See Whitehead, 'Modernising the Motherhood Archetype'.

56. See Engels, *Beyond Purdah? Women in Bengal*, p. 130.

57. *Hitavadi*, 9 April 1920, in *Report on Native Newspapers Bengal* (*RNNB*), 17 April 1920; *Dainik Basumati*, 30 March 1920, in *RNNB*, 10 April, 1920.

58. David Arnold, 'The "Discovery" of Malnutrition and Diet in Colonial India', *Indian Economic and Social History Review* 31, no. 1 (1994): 1–26.

59. Hemlata Gupta, interview, Santiniketan, 15 November 1977. Cited in Meredith Borthwick, *The Changing Role of Women in Bengal, 1849–1905* (Princeton: Princeton University Press, 1984), p. 294.

60. Manika Ray, interview, Calcutta, 14 February 1978. Cited in Borthwick, *The Changing Role of Women in Bengal*, p. 294.

61. For discussions on women's organizations, see Forbes, *Women in Modern India*; Aparna Basu and Bharati Ray, *Women's Struggle: A History of the All India Women's Conference, 1927–1990* (New Delhi: Manohar, 1990).

62. Margaret Cousins was one of the pioneers in the Irish women's suffrage movement. She came to India in 1917 at the invitation of Annie Besant. In India, Cousins worked closely with the two national women's organizations, the WIA and the AIWC. Cousins was the honorary secretary of the WIA branch of Madanapalle. Later, she edited the *Stri Dharma*, the WIA's monthly journal, launched in 1918.

63. Mary Scharlieb received her medical degree from Madras in 1875 and set up private practice there until ill health forced her to return to England, where she became a noted eugenicist active in the Infant Welfare Movement.

64. Muthulakshmi Reddi, the second president of the WIA (1933–5), the first female medical graduate of Madras Presidency, and the president of the AIWC in 1930, was born to middle-class parents in the small princely state of Pudukottah in 1886. She was the first female student to join the Madras Medical College on a state scholarship and received her medical degree with distinction in 1912. For a time, she served as house surgeon in the Government Maternity Hospital in Madras, and later she started her own private medical practice. In 1925, she went to Britain on a Government of India scholarship to specialize in diseases of women and children. A year later, Reddi became the first woman legislator in Madras when she was nominated as a member of the Legislative Council; but she resigned from this post in 1930 to protest against the imprisonment of Gandhi during the Civil Disobedience Movement. Reddi also edited *Stri Dharma*, the WIA journal, from 1931 to 1940.

65. An article published in *Stri Dharma* in 1918 pointed out that infant mortality rates in different Indian provinces compared unfavourably with those in New Zealand, where women enjoyed the right to vote since 1893. Because

of women's right to vote there, 'legislators had been compelled to improve laws relating to sanitation, the regulation of midwifery, and the purity of food which affected the health of mothers and children'. See Whitehead, 'Modernising the Motherhood Archetype', p. 197.

66. Gurusaday Dutta, *Woman of India, Being the Life of Saroj Nalini* (London: Weidenfield and Nicholson, 1929), p. 92. Also cited in Whitehead, 'Modernising the Motherhood Archetype', p. 197.

67. Balfour and Young, *The Work of Medical Women*, pp. 67–9; *Age of Consent Report 1928–29, Evidence*, pp. 67–9.

68. Saroj Nalini Dutt Memorial Association for Women's Work in Bengal, *Annual Report of the SNDMA, From the Year 1925 to 1931* (Calcutta: n.d.), pp. 2, 9.

69. 'Notun Prasuti Agar', *Banga Laksmi*, B.S. 1334–5 (1928), p. 299. Also cited in Engels, *Beyond Purdah? Women in Bengal*, p. 150.

70. For further details, see Whitehead, 'Modernising the Motherhood Archetype', p. 201.

71. See Radha Kumar, 'Organization and Struggle' in *History of Doing: An Illustrated Account of Movements for Women's Rights and feminism in India 1800–1990* (London: Verso, 1993), pp. 70–2. Cited in Ahluwalia, *Reproductive Restraints*, p. 118.

72. See Forbes, 'Women and Modernity', p. 413.

73. For discussions regarding census figures, see Leela Visaria and Pradip Visaria, 'Population', in *Cambridge Economic History of India*, vol. 2, *c. 1757 to c. 1970*, edited by Dharma Kumar and Meghnad Desai (New Delhi: Orient Longman, 1982), pp. 463–532.

74. See Barbara N. Ramusack, 'Motherhood and Medical Intervention: Women's Bodies and Professionalism in India after World War I', paper presented at the Wisconsin Conference on South Asia, Madison, Wisconsin, 1996, for discussions on baby weeks. Cited in Sujata Mukherjee, 'Disciplining the Body?'

75. See Ramusack, 'Embattled Advocates', pp. 34–64.

76. Ramusack, 'Embattled Advocates', p. 42.

77. See Ahluwalia, *Reproductive Restraints*, pp. 154–65.

78. Ahluwalia, *Reproductive Restraints*, p. 155.

79. Ruth Young, 'Medical Women and Contraception Control', *Journal of Association of Medical Women in India* 22, no. 2 (May 1934): 5–12.

80. For detailed discussions, see Ahluwalia, *Reproductive Restraints*, pp. 161–2.

81. Muthulakshmi Reddi, *AIWC Annual Reports and Conference 1932–33*, p. 90. Cited in Ahluwalia, *Reproductive Restraints*, p. 95.

82. Laxmibai Rajwade, 'Indian Mother', in Shyam Kumari Nehru, ed., *Our Cause: A Symposium by Indian Women* (Allahabad: Kitabistan, n.d.), p. 88.

83. Ahluwalia, *Reproductive Restraints*, p. 86.

84. Kamaladevi Chattopadhyaya, 'Future of Indian Women's Movement', in Nehru, *Our Cause*, p. 401.

85. See Ahluwalia, *Reproductive Restraints*, p. 91.

86. See Mukherjee, 'Disciplining the Body?', p. 204.

87. The concept of biopower, as developed by Michel Foucault in the first volume of his *History of Sexuality* (translated from the French by Robert Hurley [New York: Pantheon Books, 1978]), refers to the mechanisms employed to manage the population and discipline individuals. According to Foucault, biological life is essentially a political event: population, reproduction, and disease are central to the economic process and are, therefore, subject to political control.

88. See Mukherjee, 'Disciplining the Body?', p. 211.

89. See Guha, *Health and Population in South Asia*.

90. Mukherjee, 'Disciplining the Body?', pp. 211–12.

6 *Public Health Administration, the Famine of 1943–4, and Impact on Women*

It goes without saying that outbreak and prevalence of epidemics and endemic diseases, and availability (or non-availability) of medical relief and public health measures in general, affected levels of sickness and mortality—to varying degrees—of both male and female populations during the colonial period. Without the analyses of the gradual evolution of public health administration, outbreaks of epidemics, and the impact of the catastrophic Bengal famine of 1943–4 on women's health, any study of gender and health in colonial Bengal would remain incomplete. Therefore, this last chapter attempts to throw light on the different aspects of sickness and mortality in the pre-famine as well as in the famine period in Bengal and seeks to analyse how they were tackled. This would help to understand how far and in what ways women's health conditions were affected and specific health needs were addressed by different agencies during and after the famine years.

Recent research on issues of relationship between famine, epidemics, and mortality in colonial India has considerably enhanced our understanding of famine as an epidemiological phenomenon. The onset of famine in colonial India often resulted in the breakdown of normal social fabric and produced a series of immediate responses among victims to tackle the acute subsistence crisis, which in turn affected mortality and sickness patterns. While famine-induced starvation and migration in search of food brought about physiological decline and greater vulnerability to diseases, breakdown of social protection systems (also) often resulted in the rapid spread of sickness among the victims. The catastrophic Bengal famine of 1943 or *panchaser manvantar* (the famine of fifty, that is, of the Bengali year 1350, which corresponds to the period from mid-April 1943 through mid-April 1944) proved to be no exception. Although the causes of the famine and the extent of mortality have received much attention from different scholars,[1] several aspects of the relationship between the famine and the severe epidemics that accompanied it have remained rather under-researched.

One very important dimension of the famine–disease relationship which needs to be focused upon is whether and to what extent sickness and outbreak of epidemics were the continuation of earlier trends of pre-famine days. To be more precise, questions may be asked as to whether the famine served to accentuate pre-famine trends of malnourishment and vulnerability to diseases among certain sections of the population of colonial Bengal, and also how the specific social impacts created by the famine contributed towards the spread of sickness and epidemics. To what extent were the epidemics which accompanied the famine (and continued even after food situations were restored) a result of administrative failures? Were these policy failures (if any) a result of inherent weakness of the health care system as it had developed in pre-famine Bengal, or were they an outcome of the abnormal situations created by the famine? How did the social consequences of the famine contribute to the spread of different diseases and in what manner? Who suffered more—men or women? These are some of the issues to be addressed here. It may be mentioned that I certainly go with the argument that the famine did kill 'by adding fuel to the fire of disease and mortality present in the region'.[2]

It is also worthwhile and relevant to argue that along with long-term trends of malnutrition, endemic diseases, and the inefficiency of the public health care system which had been gradually developing in this region since the late nineteenth century, other factors like breakdown of social relations resulting in migration, vagrancy, unsanitary conditions, and absence of adequate welfare provisions during the famine also need to be taken into account to explain the level of sickness and death associated with the famine of 1943 in Bengal, particularly to understand how women were affected. Moreover, it can be pointed out that in order to assess the impact of the famine on women, the interplay of medico-social factors like prevalence of certain types of diseases affecting women resulting from the breakdown of not only public health facilities but also that of the social protection system have to be taken into account.

Poverty, Diet, Disease, and Declining Health

Since the Bengal famine of 1943 was predominantly a rural phenomenon resulting from 'a gradual collapse of the grain marketing system in early 1943'[3] rather than from any 'remarkable overall shortage of food grains in Bengal', not all sections of society and regions suffered alike.[4] Researchers have shown that although there was no remarkable shortage of food supply, declining rate of exchange entitlement of different categories of rural population due to various reasons resulted in widespread famine. Sample surveys conducted immediately after the famine threw light on the class basis of rural destitution. Karunamoy Mukerji's survey of five villages in the Faridpur district in 1944 revealed that the highest rate of proportionate destitution and death occurred among the agricultural labourers.[5] From the result of another sample survey conducted by Mahalanobis, Mukherjea, and Ghosh (1946),[6] it would appear that the most affected groups in terms of destitution were fishermen, transport workers, and agricultural workers. Undoubtedly, the Bengal famine increased the vulnerability of the rural poor, who had been suffering due to overall agricultural decline, environmental degradation, malnourishment, and diseases during the pre-famine period. In fact, throughout the nineteenth century and early twentieth century, periodic outbreaks of cholera, small pox, malaria, and plague epidemics, and attacks of other major killer diseases including influenza, kala-azar, leprosy, tuberculosis, among others, resulted in high mortality all over British India, including Bengal.

Environmental decline, agricultural deterioration of the province,[7] and dietary deficiency among the population were considered by many to be the major causes contributing to the outbreak of diseases like malaria, resulting in chronic ill health and high levels of mortality.[8]

Nineteenth-century official reports pointed out that the endemic malarious fever known as 'Burdwan fever', also referred to as 'notunjwar' by the Bengalis, which took a virulent form in the mid-nineteenth century, was caused by overpopulation, overcrowding, a diminished food supply, defective sanitary arrangements, and the silting up of rivers and water courses. Raja Digamber Mitra, the only Indian member of the official inquiry committee formed in 1863 to ascertain the causes of the extraordinary outbreak of virulent fever, emphasized the link between the transmission of malaria and the expansion of the railways and the road network. Gradually, malaria was well entrenched in the moribund region of western Bengal. C.A. Bentley, who served as the sanitary commissioner and director of public health in Bengal and wrote several monographs and pamphlets on malaria between 1907 and 1925, pointed out, 'Malaria fever is at least three times more prevalent in Western Bengal than Eastern Bengal.' He believed that the problem of malaria was linked to the problems of agricultural and environmental decline. He even suggested a temporary prohibition of embankments, which dislocated the system of natural silt irrigation and drainage.[9]

The well-known Bengali intellectual, geographer, and sociologist Radhakamal Mukherjee (1889–1966), a disciple of the Scottish environmentalist Patrick Geddes, wrote about the steady deterioration of riverine economy and agriculture in Bengal and the effects this had on the health of the people. The characteristics of the moribund delta region of western Bengal revealed that the delta-building and silt-depositing functions of Bengal's rivers had diminished in the nineteenth century. The trend continued in the early years of the twentieth century, causing massive agricultural decadence as well as the spread of malaria. Around 1935, it was pointed out that out of a total of twenty-eight districts in Bengal, seventeen were malarious. No less than 60,000 of the 86,618 villages in Bengal were affected by the disease, 'which levies an annual toll of 35,000'.[10]

The Famine Commission wrote on the impact of malaria thus: 'It lowered the capacity for work of hundreds of thousands below that of a healthy individual. Again, it tends to be worst in the season most suitable for agriculture, and sometimes the sowing and reaping of crops are seriously interfered with.' Between 1925 and 1940, malaria, cholera, and small pox accounted for more than one-third of total recorded rural deaths in Bengal. Problems like scarcity of pure drinking water, problems of adulteration of food and medicines, pollution from smoke, bad housing, and malnutrition had adverse impacts on the health of the people.[11]

It was pointed out in 1862 that the outbreak of malaria in rural Bengal had a connection with poor diets of the victims.[12] Several investigations and inquiries into diet and diseases of different segments of Bengal's population carried out from time to time actually revealed that malnourishment prevailed among a large section, which in turn led to the increasing susceptibility to disease. Under the impact of the growing importance of nutrition research in Europe in the 1860s, studies focusing on the nutritional values of different food grains of India were carried out. Rice, which was the staple food of Bengalis, was marked as being deficient in nutritional terms as compared to other Indian food grains.[13] In 1910, Captain David McCay, the Bengal sanitary commissioner, published a study on jail dietaries conducted over the previous twenty-five years. He established that the standard Bengali diet of *dal–bhat* (pulses and rice) suffered from protein deficiency. Moreover, it was also reported that there was significant inefficiency in the Bengalis' digestion of dal–bhat.[14] In the inter-War period, the newer knowledge of nutrition that developed in Britain, including the discovery of vitamins and importance of minerals[15] as well as assumptions regarding chronic ill health and susceptibility of Indians to infectious diseases, added new dimensions to the discussion on diet and malnutrition. McCarrison, the director of the Nutrition Research Laboratories at Coonoor, felt that malnutrition was the greatest problem that India had to face. He also established with experiments that the rice diet was far inferior to a 'Sikh diet' of wheat, dairy products, and meat. W.R. Aykroyd, McCarrison's successor, stressed on diet surveys of different groups of Indians, which yielded significant results.

Nationalist Indians also expressed concern about the deficiency of Bengali diets. Prafulla Chandra Ray, the first Indian professor of chemistry at the Science College of Calcutta University and the founder of the Bengal Chemical and Pharmaceutical Works,[16] observed in his evidence before the Royal Commission on Agriculture that milk deficiency in the average diet of the Bengalis led to malnutrition, stunted growth, rickets, and other such ailments.[17] In 1929, in a lecture titled 'Diet of the Bengalis' delivered to the students at Calcutta University, Chunilal Bose, the chemical examiner to the Government of Bengal and professor of chemistry at the CMC, pointed out, among other things, the 'one-sidedness' of a rice-based diet and the scarcity of milk and fish.[18] The emphasis put on the quality of foodstuff consumed, no doubt, was directed at middle-class Bengalis. For the urban and rural poor, the problem was one of not being able to consume enough quantity of staple food. In fact, as a result of widespread crop failures and scarcity in the 1930s, millions were facing the danger of starvation.[19]

Between 1935 and 1948, under the auspices of the Indian Research Funds Association, no less than 130 diet surveys were carried out in India, Burma, and Ceylon, covering 4,730 families and 21,000 individuals. These surveys were carried out in a situation that was 'normal' from the point of view of availability of food. The diet of rural groups surveyed in Bengal was found to be deficient in protective food stuff including meat, fish, fruits, and vegetables. The AIIHPH made a comparative study of dietary habits of different social groups including members from the urban professional middle class in Calcutta on the one hand and rural agriculturists in Barasat and Dinajpore on the other. The survey was based on house to house visits and covered a period of three weeks in Dinajpore and a week each in Barasat and Calcutta. The results were published in 1939 in the *IMG*. The survey revealed that the agriculturists consumed more carbohydrates derived from cereals than urban families. They derived about 80 to 90 per cent of their total calories from cereals, whereas Calcutta families derived only 48 per cent. The author finally concluded: 'The diet of the well-to-do (Calcuttans) appear to approximate in most respects to the European standards. The diet of the agriculturists is deficient in animal protein and animal fat, total calories, calcium and vitamin A.'[20]

Professor Mahalanobis, honorary secretary, Indian Statistical Institute, Calcutta, presented an analysis of the results of five different surveys of cereal consumption by various socio-economic groups in Bengal, conducted at different times between 1936 and 1942. It seemed that rural families had the highest daily rate of per capita cereal consumption. Paul Greenough has pointed out that the maximum average per capita consumption of cereals in the 1930s and 1940s (482 grams) was below the average minimum estimate (797 grams) in 1862, which would apparently mean that Bengalis suffered not only from malnutrition but undernourishment as well, which in its turn would mean increasing susceptibility to diseases and could cause considerable physical deterioration, adversely affecting recovery to normal standards of physical fitness after being attacked by diseases.

In the late 1930s and early 1940s, a number of field investigations were carried out to study morbidity patterns among villagers. One such survey was carried out by the students of the AIIHPH in 1939, in a village called Ratanpur in Hooghly district, in which malaria, diarrhoea, and dysentery were found to be the most common causes of morbidity. The survey also revealed that more than one-tenth of the population was either acutely ill or in indifferent health.[21] Poor and ill-balanced diet and malnourishment of expectant mothers had certain links with deaths from maternal causes. Data obtained by the public health department of the Government of Bengal from 1920 onwards indicated that ordinarily, 60,000 to 75,000 deaths among women were caused by prenatal, natal, and postnatal conditions. The report of 1921 mentioned that maternal causes must have been responsible for over 60,000 female deaths in Bengal during that year. It was also pointed out that pregnancy or childbirth directly or indirectly influenced deaths among females during the childbearing period to the extent of 8 to 10 per cent of those under fifteen, 50 to 60 per cent of those between fifteen and twenty, 30 to 33 per cent of those between twenty and thirty, and 3 to 4 per cent of those above forty years of age.[22]

Between 1935 and 1938, there was a steady rise in stillbirths, which showed declining maternal health.[23] In 1938, the female death rate exceeded that of males in seventeen districts in the province. Moreover, as in 1937, in 1938 too more females died than males in the age groups of five to ten and fifteen to forty years. For the female age group of fifteen to forty years, the larger mortality rate could well be attributed to greater risk due to childbirth, but the larger mortality among the age group of five to ten, which remained a uniform phenomenon over a few years, probably resulted from parental neglect of the female child, particularly when there were male children to attend to in the family.

The Government of Bengal sanctioned annual grants for facilitating dhai-training programmes. In 1932, a grant of Rs 15,000 sanctioned by the local government for the training of dhais was distributed among twenty-three district boards and twenty-five municipalities. The total number of classes conducted for the training of dhais during the year under review was 106, in which 1,212 pupil dhais were trained by 105 lecturers, all of whom were registered local medical practitioners. A total of 838 certificates and 1,060 maternity outfits were distributed to the trained dhais.[24] The Rs 15,000 sanctioned by the government for the training of dhais during the year 1938–9 was distributed among twenty-five district boards, thirty-two municipalities, the District Maternity Child Welfare Committee of the Indian Red Cross Society (Bengal Branch), Calcutta, the Saroj Nalini Dutta Memorial Association, and Barishal Baby Clinic. The total number of classes conducted for the training of dhais during 1938 was 110, in which 1,283 pupils were trained by 107 lecturers, all of whom were local medical practitioners. Excepting the training of indigenous dhais, the local government's part in maternity and child welfare work remained negligible.[25] The Public Health Report of 1940–1 mentioned that the provision for maternity services in Bengal was extremely poor, and in many rural areas such facilities did not exist at all. According to official reports, comparative neglect of the female child in a family was responsible for the prevalent high rate of tuberculosis among them.[26] Dr Crake, the health officer of Calcutta, noted that tuberculosis, which thrives in damp, dark, airless corners, played havoc in the zenanas, for lighting and ventilation were absolutely disregarded to secure privacy. The English periodical *Forward* mentioned in 1927 that the most striking feature of the disease in Calcutta was its preponderance amongst the female population. The rate of prevalence of tuberculosis among females was double of that of males.[27] An official report stated:

> Early marriage, the strain of rapid succession of pregnancies and periods of lactation and the purdah system with the inherent deprivation of fresh air and exercise which that social system involves, are all factors found to produce among the younger women of this country a great lowering of

> resistance to disease which leaves them readily susceptible to acute infections such as tuberculosis. It is not surprising that the female mortality rates are much higher than the corresponding male rates in the age groups between 15 and 40 years. Here again recorded figures leave no shadow of doubt. In Bombay city for example, out of a total of 1232 deaths from tuberculosis, 761, including 381 males and 380 females, occurred in the age groups 20 to 40 yrs. During 1931 in Calcutta 3 female deaths for every male death were recorded in the age group 10 to 15 years, 2 female deaths to one male in the group 15 to 20 years, 3 females to every male in the groups 20 to 30 years.[28]

Around 1940, the house-to-house survey carried out in Serampore revealed that the incidence of tuberculosis infection in the town was as high as 88 per cent. It was also found that the disease was predominant among girls and women between fifteen and thirty years of age.[29] Another survey in Barisal revealed that the rate of infection was higher amongst males than amongst females, but girls below ten years of age showed higher rates of infection than boys of the same age group.[30]

Coming of the Famine

Immediately before the famine, many rural areas in Bengal faced local scarcities resulting from natural disasters, pestilence, and also from wartime emergency measures which privileged urban areas. On 16 October 1942, a severe cyclone accompanied by three tidal waves hit the western districts of Bengal. The severest physical damage occurred in the southern coastal areas of Midnapur and the 24 Parganas. An estimated area of 3,200 square miles was affected, of which 450 square miles were swept by the tidal waves and around 400 square miles were wrecked by floods. 'The houses, livelihood, and property of nearly 2.5 million Bengalis were ruined or damaged by a storm that lasted less than 36 hours.'[31] Large-scale destruction of food crops, trees bearing fruits, milk cattle, and fishermen meant non-availability or scarcity of many food items in rural areas for a long period of time. The cyclone was followed by crop disease, which further ruined crops. The 'boat-denial' scheme introduced in May 1942 in many districts to counter any possible Japanese attack led to the removal or destruction of as many as 66,500 country boats, depriving poor boatmen and peasants of their sources of livelihood. The 'rice denial' scheme was another similar military measure, introduced across lower Bengal during April–May 1942, purportedly to frustrate the possible Japanese attack by allowing authorized outside agents to purchase surplus grains from cultivators. This measure severely affected the commercial exchange of grain. The war-time measures as well as natural calamities meant starvation for a large number of impoverished, rural poor. This often led to the adoption of a number of survival strategies by the victims to cope with the diminishing food supply. The onset of famine aggravated food shortage and the rural poor tried to survive by eating unusual foodstuff. The Famine Inquiry Commission pointed out, 'A high proportion of the deaths which took place in the early stages of the famine can best be described as deaths from starvation.' Many of the starving patients suffered from uncontrollable diarrhoea also known as 'famine diarrhoea', leading to rapid dehydration, weakening, and death. Starvation victims consumed large quantities of vegetables, leaves, creepers, snails, crustaceans, and subsequently even rotting or discarded food items. An interviewee in the 24 Parganas observed, 'We ate anything we could to fill the belly, except rice.'[32]

In Calcutta, the masses of rural migrant destitute were seen to eat cast-off skins of vegetables and rotten fruits collected from the streets and from around fruit stalls in markets. 'The spectacle of starving destitute ransacking refuse bins was common in Calcutta during the height of the famine.'[33] The emergency hospitals in Calcutta were filled with patients 'picked up on the streets in a state of extreme weakness and collapse, often on the point of death. They were for the most part emaciated to such a degree that the description "living skeletons" was justifiable.'[34] More or less since July 1943, the outbreak of epidemic diseases like malaria, cholera, and small pox took precedence over starvation as the main causes of the rise in mortality. Famine-induced socio-economic factors, including migration from impoverished rural areas to urban zones holding apparently better prospect for survival, breakdown of sanitary arrangements resulting from overcrowding, spread of infection, intake of unhealthy food and starvation—leading to physiological decline and collapse of resistance to diseases—and a total disintegration of the public health organization under the impact of World War II and famine led to the spread of epidemics and rise in mortality from mid-1943 onwards. 'The main poles of attraction in

1943 were the towns and cities of Bengal, where relief was known to be available, and the haven of Assam.'[35] Masses of rural destitute, mainly from the districts of 24 Parganas and Midnapore, migrated to Calcutta. Unattended dead bodies could be found lying in the streets. In October alone, 3,336 bodies had to be disposed of by relief organizations in the city.[36] It was reported from Dhaka district: 'Hindu dead bodies are being thrown into open fields, resulting in decomposition and making the atmosphere unfit for human living.' The secretary of the Manikganj Relief Committee reported:

> People attacked with cholera are lying here and there, spreading germs of diseases all over the locality, groaning in agony for days together with none to look after them.... The entire population runs the risk of being in the grip of this menace. Death is already taking heavy toll and there is no satisfactory arrangement for removal of dead bodies.[37]

(Poor) Public Health Administration

To quite a large number of people it seemed that the catastrophic famine mortality could be reduced if proper and timely administrative measures were taken for providing medical relief and arresting epidemics. At the same time, officials also maintained that public health organization suffered from certain inherent weaknesses, which had a crippling effect.

The Famine Commission observed: 'In Bengal the public health services were insufficient to meet the normal needs of the population and the level of efficiency was low. The same can of course be said of public health organization in all parts of India, but that in Bengal was below the standard of certain other provinces.'[38] The Bengal Local Self-Government Act (1885) had set up three categories of local authorities in Bengal: (*a*) the district boards (which looked after a whole district), (*b*) the local boards (in each subdivision), and (*c*) union committees (for areas within a subdivision); the last two worked under the district boards and were financially dependent on mainly district board funds. The Act empowered a district board to provide for dispensaries, hospitals, and water supply and mentioned that each district board was 'to provide so far as may be possible for the proper sanitation of each district, and to incur such expenditure or undertake such liabilities as may be necessary in that behalf'. Under section 91 of this Act, the district boards could employ sanitary inspectors who looked after rural public health works. They were placed under the supervision of the civil surgeon of the district.

The civil surgeon was responsible for anti-epidemic operations, control of vaccination and vaccination staff, and was also the adviser to the chairman of the district board with regard to public health. He was the head of medical administration of a district and supervised district hospitals and dispensaries. But he was not the executive authority in matters of public health. In 1920, a district health officer with medical qualification was appointed as the public health executive agency. He was required to perform the duties of the superintendent of vaccination. The vaccination inspectors and sub-inspectors were placed under the control and supervision of the district health officer.

By the Government of India Act, 1919 (brought into operation in 1921), public health was made a transferred subject. The department of public health and local self-government, under the charge of a minister, were responsible for public health of the entire province. The public health and hospital administration system in colonial Bengal was placed under dual control. The minister had two technical advisers who were responsible for the administration of the medical and public health departments. The former was called surgeon general and the officer-in-charge of public health was the director of public health. The department of public health consisted of two branches, namely statistical—a preventive and epidemiological side under the director of public health—and the sanitary engineering branch under the chief engineer. The functions of the director of public health were mainly advisory and not executive. Its business was to collect information as to the actual sanitary condition of the country, to investigate the incidences and causes of diseases, and to advise the government and local authorities in matters concerning the improvement of public health. It was the responsibility of the local bodies to carry out these measures.

There were four assistant directors of public health in each of the four divisions—Burdwan, Presidency, Rajshahi, and the combined divisions of Dhaka and Chittagong. The supervision of the assistant directors of public health was very ineffective; one of the biggest snags being that they were supposed to supervise district health officers who were employees of the district boards. The latter had to look after public health works in the districts. Each of the twenty-six districts had a full-time district health officer. In each health circle in the district, there were three subordinate health workers; a sanitary inspector, a health assistant, and a medicine carrier. In addition, some 100 vaccinators were appointed by the local body temporarily for about six months in the year. Public health services, water supply, hospitals, and dispensaries in the districts were financed by the local bodies. They had limited power of taxation and had to depend on grants from provincial revenues.

The provincial government itself suffered from financial stringency and was not able to provide adequate funds. The surgeon general, civil surgeons in the districts, and assistant surgeons in charge of subdivisional hospitals were in the provincial cadre and had little control over the subordinate medical staff in rural areas, who were employees of local bodies. This undoubtedly impaired the efficiency of the public health services. According to the Famine Commission, 'The general organization of the medical services and hospitals was in fact such as to render mobilization and development to meet the emergency extremely difficult.'[39]

Lack of coordination and contact among different agencies of provincial and local health organizations meant that no satisfactory attempt was made during the early months after the outbreak of the famine to deal with the situation. Brigadier Fraser, who was in charge of the military medical service during the famine, pointed out that what was found in Bengal could be described as 'either light hearted or misguided local administration'.[40] Immediately before the famine, the effects of World War II as well as natural disasters led to the spread of diseases in the provinces. With the progress of the war in Burma, numerous refugees made their escape to Bengal (or Assam). The government sent them into camps in rural areas. A large number of evacuees from Calcutta and the industrial areas took shelter in suburbs and villages in the beginning of 1942. Not only was no effort made to revamp rural health services to meet war-time needs, many public health staff were even utilized in other works including flood relief, campaigning for growing more food, and drives against hoarding of food during 1943. In reality, there was no public health organization at work in the province during that period. The withdrawal of public health staff was ordered in utter disregard of the advice given by the superior sanitary officers, which led to discontentment and a feeling of despair. The district health officer of Birbhum pointed out:

> The thana areas of Dubrajpur, Khoirasole and Rajnagore are seriously affected with cholera but my Sanitary Inspectors of these 3 thanas have been absorbed in anti-hoarding campaign and it has become almost impossible to cope with the situation by the Sanitary Assistant alone. Further, in the thana of Rampurhat sub-division both Sanitary Inspector and Sanitary Assistant have been engaged leaving the health circle to utter confusion.[41]

The outbreak of famine and the resultant mortality rate were met with a belated response from the medical department. The surgeon general pointed out in his evidence that the medical authorities at provincial headquarters did not become aware of the existence of unusual conditions until August 1943, when the sick destitute began to die in the streets of Calcutta. Lack of coordination between the provincial and district medical authorities seemed to be responsible for this.[42] According to E.W. Holland, secretary to the Government of Bengal, public health and local self-government department:

> The District Health Officers had not done as much touring as they probably ought to have. It is probably because the District Board Chairman used them for their own purposes and their tours had been rather too much dictated by the movements of the Chairman. Certainly it is true that they did not report to the Director of Public Health.[43]

Lack of finance was also responsible for the inefficiency of health services. The salaries of the members of district health services were inevitably very low and unsatisfactory. Despite war-time escalation of the cost of living, pay was not revised, which led to widespread grievances among the staff. The poor rate of travelling allowance also acted as an impediment to efficiency.

Epidemics of cholera, malaria, and small pox affected all districts of Bengal in various degrees. The reported total deaths from the cholera epidemic between July 1943 and June 1944 was 2,18,269, which was 309.7 per cent in excess of the quinquennial average for 1938–42. 'Investigations carried out in Calcutta towards the end of 1943 showed that some 40 per cent of destitute patients harboured malaria parasites.'[44] The malaria epidemic in fact broke out in famine-stricken Bengal in June 1943, peaked in December, and continued in 1944. The reported deaths from malaria in December 1943 were 202.6 per cent in excess of the quinquennial average. A small pox epidemic also broke out in severe form in December 1943, and peaked in March and April 1944.

In November 1943, although there was a clear indication of increase in cholera, no mass inoculation campaign was launched. One of the factors which contributed to the large-scale outbreak of cholera was the fact that the majority of tube wells, which were the chief sources of water supply in Bengal, had gone out of order. In all, 20,000 were out of order in the 16 districts where cholera was worst.[45] Most district boards had ineffective maintenance staff. It was decided at the public health planning conference held in November that the repair of tube wells would be the number one priority. A letter was issued by the secretary to the public health department to all district boards, stressing the importance of an immediate survey of tube wells and the need for adoption of appropriate measures for repair. Early in January 1944, the Government of Bengal sanctioned Rs 15,00,000 for improving tube wells. Work did not start until two months later and by the end of March, owing to inaction, some of the money sanctioned actually lapsed.[46] With the spread of cholera, the supply of a large amount of vaccine became the need of the hour. During the early stage of the epidemic, apart from the shortage of vaccine, the inability of the health staff to use the available vaccine affected the inoculation work. The secretary to the public health department pointed out:

> There may have been a shortage for a short period in August or September. I remember having asked the then D.P.H. in August or September why were there complaints on this score, and he told me that he was complying to the extent which he knew the District staff could use [the cholera vaccine]... He was not sending the full quantity asked for by the districts but the D.P.H. at that time reported that their demands were extravagant.[47]

Shortage of staff was another serious problem which affected the programme of inoculation. In July 1944, posts of forty-eight doctors were advertised but only ten posts could be filled.[48] The following November it was decided—because of the difficulty in obtaining qualified doctors and trained sanitary assistants—to engage untrained matriculates and give them necessary training required to perform inoculation. The appointments of sanitary inspectors were, however, delayed due to an instruction given to observe the communal ratio in recruiting them. According to many contemporaries, the outbreak of the small pox epidemic was partly due to the poor levels of vaccination among the people. In the opinion of Brigadier Fraser, 'Small pox started to occur after famine conditions had disappeared...I think it must all be attributed to a most defective vaccination campaign over a period of many years leaving a highly susceptible population behind.'[49]

According to the surgeon general of Bengal:

> If vaccination was as good as it should have been, we would not have such an attack of small pox. But it is not the fault of the vaccinators. Some of them are paid only about Rs. 10 per month and what can you expect them to do? They cannot work enthusiastically.[50]

Since there was hardly any compulsory re-vaccination, after some time, people lost their immunity from primary vaccination. The technique of vaccination might also have been, to some extent, faulty, as the under-qualified recruits had received only a brief training. Also, some of the lymph used had probably lost its potency.

It seems that unavailability of medicines in many areas was the reason for widespread prevalence of diseases. Initially, the government machinery was unable to supply sufficient quantities of quinine for free distribution to districts affected by malaria and subsequently, around November 1943, about 43,000 lbs of quinine were lying undistributed. But in December the director of public health stated that 'a vast quantity of quinine issued by the Government had gone into the black market.'[51] Thus, man-made scarcity of medicine was, to a large extent, responsible for the continuance of the malaria epidemic in rural areas in 1943. The following quote portrays the entire situation aptly:

> All the doctors in Bengal with all the quinine they could possibly get hold of, I was sure, could not have fought down the malaria and cholera epidemics that were fast decimating the people in the famine belt of the province.... High district officials (in Dacca) informed me that large quantities of quinine had arrived for distribution to hospitals and

> malaria victims in the rural areas. They were finding it a troublesome job to get hold of honest distributing agents. Doctors who signed prescriptions were corrupt sometimes, village officials to whom quinine was dispatched for local distribution were not above temptation, and the drug rarely reached, either in adequate measure or in an unadulterated form, the persons who needed it most. There was a good deal of easy money in quinine. The controlled price was about Rs. 37 a pound, and in the black market it sold at between Rs. 300/ and Rs. 400/.[52]

The epidemic situation improved gradually after an all-round effort. In November 1943, military resources were mobilized to tackle epidemics. Sixteen military hospitals throughout the province provided 2,100 beds for treatment of the sick. At the beginning of 1944, satellite treatment centres attached to rural dispensaries were also started. The Bengal Medical Relief Co-ordination Committee, a voluntary organization formed in 1944 by leading doctors and relief organizations, tried to provide medical care to the sick population of Bengal and treated more than thirteen lakh cases.

The famine of Bengal and the resultant epidemics exposed the vulnerability of the poor rural population, as well as the inefficiencies of the public health organization in Bengal. While like earlier famines of the colonial period it magnified the forces of death already present in the region, its uniqueness lay in the fact that it exposed the defects of the public health organization of colonial Bengal as well as the limitations of imperial medical policy. The quinine policy, for example, left such strong loopholes that artificial, man-made scarcity could be created to add to the woes of the famine-stricken population, which led to a tremendous rise in mortality.

Total Mortality and Age–Sex Composition

The total mortality in the Bengal famine has remained a controversial issue. The Famine Inquiry Commission pointed out: 'According to figures published by the Bengal Public Health Department, 1,873,749 people died in Bengal in 1943. The average number of deaths reported annually during the previous five years, 1938 to 1942, was 1,184,903 so that deaths in 1943 were 688,846 in excess of the quinquennial average.'[53] The commission was of the opinion that most of the famine mortality occurred between July 1943 and June 1944. It, however, pointed out that public health statistics suffered from gross inaccuracies in normal times, and records of birth as well as death, particularly in rural Bengal, suffered from under-registration as also misreporting. In fact, official reports of the late 1930s and early 1940s often unhesitatingly admitted that the system of recording vital statistics was by no means perfect or as satisfactory as it should have been. It was also mentioned time and again that the state of affairs in the rural areas was worse than in the towns because the registration of deaths and their causes were much more defective there than in urban areas.[54] In rural areas, the primary collector of mortality statistics was a village *chowkidar* (watchman) who reported to the union board office, whence by several stages the records ultimately reached the office of the director of public health. These illiterate, lowly-paid village chowkidars were ignorant of the paramount importance of vital statistics of public health.

During the famine, the chowkidars themselves were not immune from starvation and disease and some of them died, leaving their posts vacant. Many left their low-paying jobs and obtained work on military projects. Further, at the height of the famine, thousands of people left their homes and wandered across the countryside in search of food. 'Many died by the road-side—witness the skulls and bones which were to be seen there in the months following the famine. Deaths occurring in such circumstances would certainly not be recorded in the statistics of the Director of Public Health.'[55] The Famine Commission expressed the opinion that the number of deaths in excess of the average in 1943 was one million, which was 40 per cent in excess of the officially recorded mortality. It believed that collection of mortality statistics improved at the end of 1943 and so the official figure of mortality for January to June 1944 was acceptable, and thus reached the conclusion that 'about 1.5 million deaths occurred as a direct result of the famine and epidemics which followed in its train.'

Various other estimates of famine mortality also exist. One of the most widely published contemporary unofficial estimates was presented by Professor K.P. Chattopadhyay, from the department of anthropology at the Calcutta University. Based on a sample survey of some of the worst-hit areas, covering more than 800 family units with a total membership of more than 3,800 during June–December 1943, Professor Chattopadhyay's estimate calculated the total mortality to be around 3.5 million. Later, however, Chattopadhyay himself revised the estimate and proposed a figure of 2.7 million as a minimum estimate.[56] The figures presented by the Famine Commission and Chattopadhyay have been criticized by many; the former being criticized for arbitrariness of the correction factor and the latter for poor selection of sample and the lack of evidence in favour of the projection of the sample onto the entire population. Amartya Sen has suggested that the famine mortality actually extended far beyond June 1944, and accordingly presented a revised estimate of three million famine deaths over the period 1943–6.[57] Paul Greenough has proposed that the excess mortality due to the famine during 1943–6 would be somewhere between 3.5 and 3.8 million. This calculation is partly based on the unpublished data collected by a group of researchers of the Indian Statistical Institute (led by Professor P.C. Mahalanobis), which carried out a sample survey of 13,358 households in 40 of Bengal's 86 subdivisions around 1946.[58]

The age–sex composition of famine mortality has also come under close scrutiny. The general trend in the age composition in famine mortality in Bengal seemed to conform to earlier famine experiences. While deaths of infants below one year decreased, the proportion remained the same for children below five in average mortality in pre-famine days and in excess mortality in the famine year. The mortality in proportion of deaths for old people over sixty was high, just as it used to be in the pre-famine days.[59] In many of the late nineteenth- and early twentieth-century Indian famines, infants below one year appeared to have experienced a relative advantage in terms of proportional rise in death compared to children and adults. For example, during the famine of 1876–8 in Madras, Bombay, and United Provinces, mortality rates for infants increased proportionately by a smaller amount in the peak mortality year than for other groups of children. This seems to be consistent with the hypothesis that infants are rather better protected than children during acute food crisis.[60] It is generally argued that the age–sex composition of mortality effects of a famine is an outcome of two factors, namely physiological vulnerability and social protection. In analysing the impact of famine on infant mortality, a distinction can be made between the effects of 'prenatal exposure' and 'postnatal exposure'. While the former works through maternal nutritional stress and associated maternal infections, the latter generally includes nutritional deficiency of the infants, poor care, and so forth. Many neonatal deaths in poor countries like India are due to chronic maternal malnutrition, tetanus, and inadequate perinatal care. These factors seem most unlikely to be influenced by acute events such as famine.[61] Moreover, infants might be expected to be relatively better protected from extreme mortality during famine as they depend on breast milk, an infant's ideal form of nutrition. It seems that young children are comparatively physiologically more vulnerable to nutritional deficiency associated with famine as they, in their period of growth, have small reserves of nutrients and energy. The effect of famine on young children's mortality rate could either be lessened or be heightened depending on the cultural practices prevalent in the society struck by acute subsistence crisis. The vulnerability of young children during acute food shortage may be offset by cultural norms which might influence intra-household food distribution in their favour. Conversely, children's condition may worsen and vulnerability might increase during subsistence crisis due to the existence of cultural rules which favour active, adult males within the family to get the larger share of scarce family resources first, and other members eat whatever is left afterwards. It has been pointed out that '(t)he history of famines over the world is full of gruesome stories of neglect, abandonment, sale, or even murder of children'.[62]

It is also true that children are possibly worst hit by the breakdown of family ties, which seems to be a very common commitment of famines. Das's sample survey of destitute in Calcutta suggested that more than 20 per cent of the street destitute were children who had separated from their parents or parents who had abandoned all their children.[63]

Male–Female Mortality

It must be kept in mind that like total mortality, the sex composition of victims of famine-induced epidemics has also remained a debatable issue. One general assumption, which sometimes appeared in official famine reports in colonial India, was that women were more resilient than men during times of disasters like famines. Sir Charles Elliot, famine commissioner of Mysore in 1876 and census commissioner of India for the 1881 census, pointed out, 'all the authorities seem agreed that women succumb to famine less easily than men.'[64]

In case of the Bengal Famine of 1943 also, the Famine Inquiry Commission reported that in 1943 there was a higher proportion of increase in male deaths compared to female deaths.[65] According to the commission, this seemed to conform to the general trend of mortality in Bengal. The commission noted: 'Actually more male than female deaths are normally reported in Bengal, which is due to the higher proportion of males in the population, & to the excess of male births (108 male to 100 female), which leads to more deaths among infants of the male sex.' A sample survey carried out in rural areas by T.C. Das, lecturer in social anthropology at the Calcutta University, investigated 4,833 deaths, of which 56.7 per cent were male and 42.3 per cent female. Apparently, various famine hospital records showed the same trend. The commission also referred to the different picture presented by another investigation made by Professor P.C. Mahalanobis, which covered 2,622 families residing in villages in 7 subdivisions of Bengal. The overall mortality among females in these groups as a whole was higher than among males. The commission remarked: 'There was, however, considerable irregularity in the proportionate sex mortality in the various sub-divisions, & in some sub-divisions the male mortality, on a percentage basis, exceeded the female. The aggregate figures are influenced by the data from one sub-division in which, for some reason, female deaths greatly exceeded male deaths.'[66]

Amartya Sen has challenged the view that mortality among men was higher than women. On the basis of the Census of India 1951, he has shown that the male population exceeded the female population in Bengal, and the recorded death rate per unit of population was higher for women in every year during the decade 1941–50, through the famine.[67]

Did Women Suffer More Than Men?

While there are controversies regarding issues like total mortality and age–sex composition of famine victims, there is no doubt that women suffered more than men because of abandonment and destitution, leading to the adoption of survival strategies which affected health status.

Sometimes female victims seemed to receive less relief than their male counterparts, which no doubt contributed/added to their difficulty. Based on data furnished by the Bengal Relief Committee (BRC), Paul Greenough made an analysis of the characteristics of different households receiving relief (food, medicine, and clothing) between October 1943 and June 1946, to show that males accounted for more than 60 per cent of the total recipients.[68]

The sample survey undertaken by Professor Mahalanobis and others in 1946 pointed out that in January 1943 the destitute in Bengal numbered around 7.5 lakhs; between January 1943 and May 1944, there was a further increase of about 3.3 lakhs in the numbers of the destitute. Pre-famine poor health and economic status of the victims aggravated destitution and disease.

The worst-affected sections of the population due to destitution comprised mainly the very young, the old and infirm, and women.[69] Immediately before the famine, many rural areas in Bengal faced local scarcities resulting from natural disasters, pestilence, and also war-time emergency measures. In rural Bengal, where women customarily had a low socio-economic status, crises associated with war and famine aggravated their limited access to food and other essential requirements. The onset of famine led to the adoption of a number of survival strategies by the victims to cope with diminishing supply of food.

The priorities of the family often used to be pro-male in distress situations. There were cultural imperatives also—as shown by Paul Greenough in his study—which dictated survival of the male over the female. This hastened the problem of large-scale destitution among women. When it became difficult to make both ends meet in 1943, rural families abandoned their non-earning members. At the onset of the conditions of scarcity, adult men left villages and sought temporary work at the military construction sites. Starvation drove thousands of people from villages to nearby towns and far-flung cities. Travails of this nature caused the break-up of families. The male 'providers' failed to provide for the dependents in 1943–4; and adult males abandoned women and children in large numbers. Sickness, unemployment, desertion, and death of male earners in the family were some of the basic reasons for the large proportion of destitute women.[70] A survey of 2,537 persons randomly selected from among the destitute residing in the streets of Calcutta in September 1943 revealed that 47.3 per cent were male and 52.7 per cent women. When asked what compelled them to leave their villages and come to Calcutta, the women answered that they were asked by their husbands to go elsewhere to search for food. Some women also said that they were deserted by their husbands who failed to maintain them.[71]

The famine victimized women in other ways too. Shortage of cloth curtailed women's mobility and led to humiliation. F.O. Bell, a civil servant, who was making a tour of rural areas during the famine, found that women were 'badly off for clothing as the people who used to help them are badly off'.[72]

Poverty, hunger, destitution, abandonment by male members of the family, and also the need to provide for other family members—particularly the young—often pushed women into the flesh trade in the absence of alternative means of survival. Prostitution became rampant, mostly near cantonment areas. It was pointed out: 'A section of the contractors has made a profession of selling the girls to the military. There are places in Chittagong, Camilla and Noakhali where women sold themselves literally in hordes, and young boys act as pimps for the military.'[73]

Purchase of girl-children by networks of prostitutes for future sexual exploitation was also reported in the press.[74] According to an estimate made by P.C. Joshi in 1944, out of 1,25,000 destitute women in Calcutta, nearly 30,000 were in brothels, and one in four was a young girl.[75] Different anecdotes also depict how distress and famine forced poor women to join the Military Labour Corps where they were infected by venereal diseases.[76]

The reports on the health of the army in India indicated a steady increase in venereal diseases from 1938 to 1944. The official view never recognized how, since the beginning of the war, increased troop movement in Calcutta and the interiors of Bengal had contributed to the rising level of prostitution and the subsequent spread of venereal diseases among these unfortunate women.

According to the estimates of local medical practitioners, in the famine-affected regions, nearly 5–10 per cent of the population were victims of venereal diseases.[77] In government clinics, the attendance of patients suffering from venereal diseases increased remarkably between January and August 1944. Due to the absence of medical centres in the remote districts that were reporting these cases, it was hard to bring the situation under control.

From late 1943 onwards, different women's organizations of Bengal such as the All Bengal Women's Self-Defence Committee, the AIWC, and the Nari Sewa Samiti drew attention to the increasing menace of sexually transmitted diseases and criticized the government for its negligence of the problem. In its 1944 session, the AIWC resolved that '(a) exemplary punishment be meted out to the culprits [those who forced women into prostitution] by official authorities; (b) recognised organizations take immediate steps for the protection and rehabilitation of such women [who became the victims of the flesh trade]; and (c) government by legislative and executive action safeguard their [women suffering from venereal diseases] interests'.[78]

The year 1944 also witnessed another significant adverse effect of the famine—a sharp decline in child birth. This could perhaps be explained by several complex factors like decrease in marital intercourse because of separation, deliberate birth control or self-restraint, stillbirths, abortions, and even physiological changes because of starvation, which are known to render women infertile. As pointed out by Paul Greenough, since child-bearing was a hazardous process, a lower rate of birth seemed to contribute to increased chances of survival of women of reproductive age in famine-affected Bengal.[79]

Later on, when the government drew up a twenty-year plan of post-war reconstruction in 1944 and planned anti-malaria drives, it ignored problems related to venereal diseases. It is, however, noteworthy that the Bhore Committee or the Health Survey and Development Committee, which was set up in the same year, declared in its report (1946) that 'any plan for improving the health of the community must pay special attention to the development of measures for adequate health protection to mothers and children'.[80]

In its final report, the Famine Inquiry Commission had also pointed out earlier that dietary deficiency among Indians, particularly among women and children, was responsible for much ill health. Thus, we notice the articulation of a spirit of criticism and concern in official expressions regarding welfare works in the sphere of maternal and child health, which had earlier remained at the margins of public health concerns. Remarkably, demands for women's health improvement also became part and parcel of anticolonial organizational politics of middle-class women.

Notes and References

1. Two excellent studies on the Bengal famine are Paul R. Greenough, *Prosperity and Misery in Modern Bengal: The Famine of 1943–1944* (New York: Oxford University Press, 1982); and Amartya Sen, *Poverty and Famines: An Essay on Entitlement and Deprivation* (New Delhi: Oxford University Press, 1984). Among other notable works on famines in the colonial era are: Malavika Mukherjee, *The Famine of 1896–1897 in Bengal: Availability or Entitlement Crisis?* (New Delhi: Orient Longman, 2004); Ramesh Chandra Dutta, *Indian Famines: Their Cause and Prevention* (London: P.S. King, 1901); B.M. Bhatia, *Famines in India: A Study in Some Aspects of the Economic History of India, 1860–1965*, 2nd edition (Bombay: Asia Publishing House, 1967); Srimanjari, *Through War and Famine Bengal, 1939–45* (New Delhi: Orient BlackSwan, 2009); Madhusree Mukerjee, *Churchill's Secret War: The British Empire and the Ravaging of India during World War II* (New York: Basic Books, 2010).

2. A.K. Sen, '*Famine Mortality: A Study of the Bengal Famine of 1943*', in *Peasants in History: Essays in Honour of Daniel Thorner*, edited by E.J. Hobsbawm, W. Kula, Ashok Mitra, K.N. Raj, and Ignacy Sachs (Calcutta: Oxford University Press, 1980), pp. 194–220. Cited in David Arnold, 'Social Crisis and Epidemic Disease in the Famines of Nineteenth Century India', *Social History of Medicine* 6, no. 3 (1993): 385–404.

3. Greenough, *Prosperity and Misery in Modern Bengal*, p. 85.

4. A. Sen, *Poverty and Famines*, p. 63.

5. Karunamoy Mukerji, *Agriculture, Famine and Rehabilitation in South Asia* (Santiniketan: Visva Bharati, 1965).

6. P.C. Mahalanobis, R. Mukherjea, and A. Ghosh, *A Sample Survey of After-effects of the Bengal Famine of 1943* (Calcutta: Statistical Publishing Society, 1946).

7. Some of the major works on agriculture in Bengal in the colonial period include the following: Sugata Bose, *Agrarian Bengal: Economy, Social Structure and Politics, 1919–47* (Cambridge: Cambridge University Press, 1986); Partha Chatterjee, *Bengal, 1920–47: The Land Question* (Calcutta: K.P. Bagchi & Co., 1984); Asok Sen, Partha Chatterjee, and Saugata Mukherji, eds, *Three Studies on the Agrarian Structure in Bengal, 1840–1947* (New Delhi: Oxford University Press, 1982); B.B. Chaudhuri, 'Agricultural Production In Bengal and Bihar, Coexistence of Decline and Growth, 1859–1885', *Bengal: Past and Present* 88, part 2, no. 166 (July–December 1969); B.B. Chaudhuri, 'Growth of Commercial

Agriculture in Bengal, 1859–1885', *Indian Economic and Social History Review* 7 (March–June 1970): 25–60; B.B. Chaudhuri, 'The Process of Depeasantisation in Bengal and Bihar, 1885–1947', *Indian Historical Review* 2, no. 1 (July 1975): 105–65; M. Mufakharul Islam, *Bengal Agriculture, 1920–1946* (Cambridge: Cambridge University Press, 1978).

8. For details on malaria see Arabinda Samanta, *Malarial Fever in Colonial Bengal, 1820–1939: Social History of An Epidemic* (Kolkata: Firma KLM Private Limited, 2002); Ihtesham Kazi, 'Environmental Factors Contributing To Malaria in Colonial Bengal', in *Disease and Medicine in India: A Historical Overview*, edited by Deepak Kumar (New Delhi: Tulika, 2001), pp. 123–31; Ira Klein, 'Malaria and Mortality in Bengal, 1840–1921', *Indian Economic and Social History Review* 9, no. 2 (June 1972): 132–60; Sujata Mukherjee, 'Environmental Thoughts and Malaria in Colonial Bengal: A Study in Social Response', *Economic and Political Weekly* 43, nos 12–13 (2008): 54–61; Rohan Deb Roy, '"An Awful, Unseen Visitant": The Return of Burdwan Fever', *Economic and Political Weekly* 43, nos 12–13 (2008): 62–70.

9. Bentley began investigating the causes of malaria in Bengal from the following basic premise:

> The phenomenon of epidemic disease is always the result of a change in environment. Investigation of diseases and epidemics, whether of malaria, plague, cholera, and other infective disease becomes essentially a study of man's relationship to his environment of which parasites form only a part.... It follows that the investigation of the causes of malaria disease among a population, necessitates a consideration not only of the parasites of malaria and anopheline carriers which may represent only one factor in the condition, but an inquiry into every detail of human environment.... The whole question of rural malaria in India, is bound up with the problem of agriculture.... The attempt to reduce malaria by such measures as drainage or the clearing of jungle unless accompanied by an extension and improvement in cultivation is foredoomed to failure.

For a discussion of his works, see Sujata Mukherjee, 'Malaria and Morbidity in Colonial Bengal', in *The Imperial Embrace: Society and Polity under the Raj: Essays in Honour of Sunil Kumar Sen*, edited by Ranjit Kumar Roy (Calcutta: Rabindra Bharati University, 1993).

10. For details, see Radhakamal Mukherjee, *The Changing Face of Bengal: A Study in the Riverine Economy*, with an introduction by Arun Bandopadhyay (Calcutta: University of Calcutta, reprint, 2008–9).

11. For detailed discussions, see Kabita Ray, *History of Public Health: Colonial Bengal 1921–1947* (Calcutta: K.P. Bagchi & Company, 1998).

12. See B.B. Chaudhuri, 'Agrarian Economy and Agrarian Relations in Bengal, 1859–85', in *History of Bengal, 1757–1905*, edited by N.K. Sinha (Calcutta: University of Calcutta, second edition, 1996).

13. David Arnold, 'The "Discovery" of Malnutrition and Diet in Colonial India', *Indian Economic and Social History Review* 31, no. 1 (1994): 1–26.

14. India, Sanitary Commissioner (Bengal), *Investigations on Bengal Jail Dietaries with Some Observations on the Influence of the Dietary on the Physical Development and Well-Being of the People of Bengal* (Calcutta: Superintendent of Government Printing, 1910). Cited in Greenough, *Prosperity and Misery in Modern Bengal*, pp. 74–5.

15. For details, see Michael Worboys, 'The Discovery of Colonial Malnutrition between the Wars', in *Imperial Medicine and Indigenous Societies*, edited by David Arnold (Manchester: Manchester University Press, 1988), pp. 208–25.

16. For details on P.C. Ray, see Pratik Chakrabarti, *Western Science in Modern India: Metropolitan Methods, Colonial Practices* (New Delhi: Permanent Black, 2004); J. Lourdusamy, *Science and National Consciousness in Bengal (1870–1930)* (New Delhi: Orient Longman, 2004).

17. *Report of the Royal Commission on Agriculture, 1926–28*, vol. 4, p. 381.

18. Chunilal Bose, 'Diet of the Bengalis', in his *Food: The Adharchandra Mookerjee Lectures for 1929* (Calcutta: University of Calcutta, 1930), pp. 92–110.

19. See Greenough, *Prosperity and Misery in Modern Bengal*, p. 70.

20. Durgadas Mitra, 'Diet and Nutrition of Bengali Hindus', *Indian Medical Gazette* (April 1939), p. 229.

21. 'The Health Status of a Bengali Village: All India Institute of Hygiene and Public Health Students' Survey', *Indian Medical Gazette* (June 1942).

22. *54th Annual Report of the Director of Public Health for Bengal, 1921*, available at the National Library, Kolkata.

23. The provincial figures for four years are provided below to show that stillbirths were steadily increasing from year to year:

1935: 72,558

1936: 73,399

1937: 77,623

(*The Report of the Director of Public Health, Bengal, for the Year 1938*, available at the National Library, Kolkata.)

24. Government of Bengal (GoB), Public Health Department, *Bengal Public Health Report for the Year 1932*.

25. Government of Bengal, Public Health Department, *Bengal Public Health Report for the Year 1938.*

26. K. Ray, *History of Public Health*, p. 75n143.

27. 'Toll of Epidemics in Calcutta', *Forward*, 28 August 1927, p. 18, cited in K. Ray, *History of Public Health*, p. 75n142.

28. *Annual Report of the Public Health Commissioner with the Government of India for 1932*, vol. 1, section II.

29. *Bengal Public Health Report for the Year 1942*, p. 14.

30. *Bengal Public Health Report for the Year 1942*, p. 14.

31. *Bengal Legislative Assembly Proceedings*, 64:3, March 1943, pp. 212–13; 65:1, July 1943, pp. 251–3. Cited in Greenough, *Prosperity and Misery in Modern Bengal*, p. 93.

32. Greenough, *Prosperity and Misery in Modern Bengal*, p. 231.

33. John Woodhead, *Famine Inquiry Commission: Report on Bengal* (Delhi: Manager of Publications, 1945), p. 117.

34. Woodhead, *Famine Inquiry Commission*, p. 116.

35. Woodhead, *Famine Inquiry Commission*, pp. 143–4.

36. K.C. Ghosh, *Famines in Bengal: 1770–1943* (Calcutta: Indian Associated Publishing, 1944), pp. 119–20. Cited by A. Sen, *Poverty and Famines*, p. 57.

37. Greenough, *Prosperity and Misery in Modern Bengal*, p. 164.

38. Woodhead, *Famine Inquiry Commission*, p. 132.

39. Woodhead, *Famine Inquiry Commission*, p. 135.

40. *Nanavati Papers, Memoranda and Oral Proceedings of the Famine Commission, 1944–1945* (National Archives of India, New Delhi), vol. 2, p. 496.

41. *Nanavati Papers*, vol. 2, p. 237.

42. Woodhead, *Famine Inquiry Commission*, p. 135.

43. Nanavati *Papers*, vol. 3, p. 703.

44. Woodhead, *Famine Inquiry Commission*, p. 116.

45. *Nanavati Papers*, vol. 3, p. 710.

46. *Nanavati Papers*, vol. 2, p. 386.

47. *Nanavati Papers*, vol. 2, p. 386.

48. *Nanavati Papers*, vol. 3, p. 710.

49. *Nanavati Papers*, vol. 2, p. 497.

50. Indian Historical Records Commission, *Proceedings of the Session*, vol. 56 (Superintendent Government Printing, India, 1997), p. 93.

51. Woodhead, *Famine Inquiry Commission*, p. 138.

52. T.G. Narayan, *Famine over Bengal* (Calcutta: The Book Company Limited, 1944), pp. 184, 186, 189. Cited in Greenough, *Prosperity and Misery in Bengal*, p. 170.

53. Woodhead, *Famine Inquiry Commission*, p. 108.

54. In India, including Bengal, the system of registration of vital statistics underwent many changes. In February 1868, the Government of Bengal issued orders for procuring 'mortuary returns' through municipalities, and through village chowkidars and police from non-municipal areas. In 1897, the Bengal Births and Deaths Registration Act of 1873 was extended to all municipal towns and subsequently, in 1926, to all the district board areas.

55. Woodhead, *Famine Inquiry Commission*, p. 109.

56. A. Sen, *Poverty and Famines*, p. 197; Greenough, *Prosperity and Misery in Bengal*, pp. 300–1.

57. A. Sen, *Poverty and Famines*, p. 202.

58. Greenough, *Prosperity and Misery in Bengal*, pp. 299–315.

59. A. Sen, *Poverty and Famines*, p. 213.

60. Arup Maharatna, 'Infant and Child Mortality during Famines in Late 19th and Early 20th Century India', *Economic and Political Weekly* (July 1996): 1777.

61. L.C. Chen and A.K.M.A Chowdhury, 'Dynamics of Contemporary Famine', *International Population Conference*, Mexico, vol. 1. Cited in Maharatna, 'Infant and Child Mortality', p. 1783.

62. Maharatna, 'Infant and Child Mortality', p. 1776.

63. Tarak Chandra Das, *Bengal Famine (1943), As Revealed in a Survey of the Destitute in Calcutta* (Calcutta: University of Calcutta, 1949), p. 86.

64. For this and other observations, see *Census of India 1911*, vol. 1, part I, appendix to Chapter 6; and also T.C. Das, *Bengal Famine*, pp. 93–6. Cited in A. Sen, *Poverty and Famines*, pp. 210–11.

65. Famine Inquiry Commission, India (1945a), pp. 110–11. Cited in A. Sen, *Poverty and Famines*, p. 211.

66. Woodhead, *Famine Inquiry Commission*, p. 111.

67. *Census of India 1951*, vol. 6, part IB, tables 7 and 8, pp. 29–30. Cited in A. Sen, *Poverty and Famines*, p. 211.

68. Greenough, *Prosperity and Misery in Bengal*, pp. 184–90.

69. Srimanjari, *Through War and Famine Bengal*, p. 209n53.

70. See Greenough, *Prosperity and Misery in Bengal*, Chapter 5.

71. T.C. Das, *Bengal Famine*. Cited in Greenough, *Prosperity and Misery in Bengal*, p. 220.

72. F.O. Bell, *F.O. Bell Papers*, 28 September 1944. Cited in Sreemanjari, *Through War and Famine Bengal*, p. 199.

73. Bhowani Sen, *Rural Bengal in Ruins*, translated by N. Chakravarty (Bombay: People's Publishing House, 1945), pp. 29–30.

74. Greenough, *Prosperity and Misery in Bengal*, p. 223.

75. Renu Chakravarty, *Communists in Indian Women's Movement: 1940–50* (New Delhi: Peoples' Publishing House, 1980), p. 43.

76. It was recorded:

> In Chittagong, women from the families of fishermen, scavengers and others were forced by the distress in the wake of the famine to join the Military Labour Corps in large numbers. From there, many came back infected with venereal diseases. This is true not only of Chittagong; in many famine-devastated areas of Bengal, womanhood has been dishonoured.

(B. Sen, *Rural Bengal in Ruins*, pp. 29–30. Cited in Greenough, *Prosperity and Misery in Bengal*, p. 178).

77. P.G. Bhaduri, *Aftermath of Bengal Famine: Problem of Rehabilitation and Our Task* (Calcutta: 1945), pp. 31–2. Cited in Sreemanjari, *Through War and Famine Bengal*, p. 205n42.

78. Srimanjari, *Through War and Famine Bengal*, p. 205n41.

79. See Greenough, *Prosperity and Misery in Bengal*, pp. 309–15.

80. See David Arnold, 'Official Attitudes to Population, Birth Control and Reproductive Health in India, 1921–1946', in *Reproductive Health in India: History, Politics, Controversies*, edited by Sara Hodges (New Delhi: Orient Longman, 2006).

Epilogue

The Health Survey and Development Committee, chaired by Sir Joseph Bhore (a high-ranking Indian Civil Service officer), was set up by the Government of India towards the end of the war in 1944. The Committee consisted of twenty-five members and included three women—Dr H.M. Lazarus, chief medical officer of the WMS, Dr D.J.R. Dadabhoy, a former president of the Association of Medical Women in India, and Mrs K. Shuffi Tyabji. Drawing on the findings of the Central Advisory Board's special committee of 1938, it concluded that the extent of maternal mortality had been greatly underestimated and that in British India maternal deaths numbered over 2,00,000 annually.

In its report presented in 1946, the committee presented a critique of the relative neglect of women's health in the past and made a strong plea for improved facilities in the future. Drawing attention to the fact that annually nearly four million women suffered varying degrees of disability and discomfort as a result of childbearing, the committee declared that 'any plan for improving the health of the community must pay special attention to the development of measures for adequate health protection to mothers and children.'[1]

In its report, the Bhore Committee also noted that there was no evidence of recognition of the need of an organized programme in the field of maternal and child welfare by governments, and the growth in this field occurred only through voluntary effort. Notwithstanding the fact that state support for health care for women was far from adequate and rather underdeveloped, the significance of different developments in the field of women and medicine lay elsewhere.

As pointed out earlier, colonial medical discourse and practice in nineteenth-century-British India, no doubt, eventually privileged Western medicine based on knowledge of human anatomy gathered from dissection over indigenous medical systems. As the nineteenth century progressed and Western medicine received patronage from the rulers, education in scientific medicine and its dissemination were regarded as a cornerstone of the civilizing mission, and underscored the colonizers' cultural authority. It meant that the domain of traditional medicine (and of traditional caregivers) was gradually discredited and marginalized in official medical policies. Along with the growth and development of hospital medicine in the course of the nineteenth century, traditional healing practice was castigated as unscientific and inadequate in the colonial rhetoric. Apparently, the construction of lying-in hospitals and maternity wards in different hospitals had the humanitarian goal of saving mothers' and children's lives. At the same time, this was meant to serve a political agenda. The aim was to win support from an enlightened public as well as from bureaucrats, who were convinced that a large and healthy population was the basis for the economic, fiscal, and military strength of states. This kind of reasoning helped to make available public money for founding lying-in hospitals during the second half of the eighteenth century. Moreover, maternity hospitals were critically needed in order to provide practical clinical training alongside theoretical instruction. Thus, it served the purpose of providing practical training to medical students.

While traditional medical care played an important role for a large section of male as well as female population, a clamour for the expansion and modernization of female health care by applying biomedicine became an inextricable part of the history of institutionalization of curative medicine in the colonial period. Undoubtedly, the transition from bedside medicine to hospital medicine meant that a space was created—through the institutionalization of Western therapies—for the legitimization of medical intervention over individual female (as well as male) bodies. As an avenue was opened for medical intervention into female bodies, it also helped the growth of gynaecological knowledge. The latter, in its turn, (re)enforced—to some extent—gender, class, and racial hierarchies.

Physiological discussions and theorization regarding the woman's body since the mid-nineteenth century were aided by pathological specimens in the Museum of the CMC. In his book *Pathologica Indica* published in 1848, Allan Webb, the curator of the Museum of the Calcutta Medical College, noted the morbid state of the sexual and reproductive organs of native women. According to Webb, Indian women did not menstruate earlier than twelve years unless 'unnaturally forced' by mechanical or mental stimulation.[2] He also tried to explain the cause of abortion among the Hindu population and pointed out that attractive young wives of polygamous, ageing *kulin* Brahmin grooms, who became widows soon after marriage, were lured into illegitimate sexual liaisons. In their attempts to get rid of the unwanted pregnancies, the Hindus, 'more than any other race', indulged in foeticide. It was perceived to be a cultural phenomenon, without a natural, biological, or climatic basis, which could be reformed as well. This liberal, racialist discourse on puberty seemed to bolster imperial confidence in the reform of native women's bodies.

John Roberton, a Manchester surgeon, also expressed more or less similar views. He published a few articles in the 1840s in the *Edinburgh Medical and Surgical Journal* on the subject of menstruation among 'Hindus', 'Negroes', and 'Esquimaux', which were later published in the form of a book.[3] According to him, not climate but social customs and cultural practices such as early marriages, precocity, men refusing to eat with women, polygamy, the treatment of widows, lack of education and other such factors were responsible for creating divergence among races, which had a bearing on women's bodies. Roberton argued that women's menstrual cycle in different parts of the globe could give an indication of racial difference. He concluded:

> The difference between the European and the Hindu...must be sought in race, for if the early menstruation of tropical women was found to be

> a natural fact, then their inferiority is determined; and it will be in vain, by means of the missionary, of education, or of enlightened legislation, to attempt the reversal of laws based on physiological difference.[4]

Roberton based his observations on sources like Mounstuart Elphinstone's *History of India*, W. Adam's *Adam's Reports on Vernacular Education in Bengal and Behar*, N.B. Halhed's *A Code of Gentoo Laws*, and Allan Webb's *Pathologica Indica*. Dr Gooddeve, professor of midwifery at the CMC, helped him with statistics on puberty. Dr Gooddeve cited ninety cases of Hindu women and the average age of menarche was established as twelve years, whereas the average age for English women was established as fourteen years based on the evidence collected from 2,169 cases.[5]

Gooddeve collected evidence from Madhusudan Gupta, who was originally a teacher of the Native Medical Institution. Madhusudan Gupta, in his evidence before the Fever Hospital Committee, pointed out that Hindu women 'are not so subject to some of the diseases I have mentioned as the males...but they are very subject to hysteria, and irregularities of the menses'.[6] He described how the post-partum Bengali woman, who was considered impure, was placed in a dark and damp room with very poor ventilation and suffered from fever, pain in the belly, headache and giddiness, and other such ailments because of unhygienic circumstances. According to him,

> The harm done to the public health by such customs is permanent and absolute...for children too suffer, by being kept in the same smoky room, the treatment of the mother had bad effects upon her milk, and this also disorders the child...I do not see in the town of Calcutta any children who are of perfect health.[7]

Long after Madhusudan's statements, in a treatise on motherhood, which was 'lovingly given over to the hands of the educated women of Bengal', Gunga Prasad Mukhopadhyaya, the author, presented (like many other texts of this period) a critique of the unhygienic condition of the *sutikaghar*, including the inadequate ventilation and filthy practices of midwives. In the second part of the book, the author advised on how to take care of the infant. The basic underpinnings were the idea of the cultivation of an improved, sanitary way of birth management for bhadralok society, which was differentiated from the primitive, lower-caste ways of non-modern birthing and infant care.

By the second half of the nineteenth century, the class basis of sanitary citizenship was evidently formulated. The author chided the bhadramahila for spending her time reading only for pleasure, and urged them instead to self-educate themselves in the management of pregnancy, preservation of sanitation and hygiene in the sutikagriha, and also in raising the child. The activities of the lower-caste dhai—regarded as primitive, unhygienic practices—were to be constantly supervised and regulated. Thus the 'modern woman' came into being with the marginalization of traditional and popular knowledge, and by distancing their class from women of the lower classes and castes.[8] It has been pointed out rightly that the corpus of writing on the medicalization of childbirth and childcare, including *Matrisiksha,* formed part of a distinctive genre of writings that aimed at the care of the self, the cultivation of sanitary virtues, and also the management of racial futures.[9] Undoubtedly, 'in this prose of sanitary citizenship, racial and caste differences were preserved, reiterated and rearticulated as class by an urban, modern, upper class.'[10] Discussions regarding sutikaghar also 'shed light on the extended meanings of public health in the late nineteenth century, and the dynamic interaction of race, class and gender in the definition of sanitary citizenship and the Bengali modern.'[11]

The colonial state sought to represent itself as an agent of modernity in India, particularly as this related to 'improving' Indian women's health. Yet it showed hesitation in fulfilling the agenda it set out for itself. It has to be remembered that the colonial administrative structure and its discourse were shaped by heterogeneous perspectives. There was no administrative homogeneity; different colonial authorities articulated competing visions of the role assigned to the state in furthering and supporting the spread of health education—including contraceptive information—in the late colonial period. In their hesitation to support the cause of birth control, some argued that they feared the colonial state would be acting against the sensibilities of Indians if it officially endorsed and supported wider dissemination of contraceptive information. There appeared to be a division on the question of whether India qualified as an 'over-populated' country. Many saw the demographic problem not so much as one of sheer numbers but one of eugenics, where the birth rates of the 'desirable' social, economic, and cultural elites were lower than those of the prolific subaltern orders.

During the 1920s, 1930s, and 1940s the colonial state was reluctant to advocate reform policies that it feared might alienate the more conservative elements within Indian society. In 1929, the Age of Consent Committee received greater support from Indian women's organizations than from the colonial state, which was very reluctant to raise either the age of marriage or the age of sexual consent within marriages for Indian women, given the strong opposition to the 1891 Age of Consent Act. In the Council of State debates, the government representatives were unwilling to defend the demand for state support of birth control, even when it was framed as a health issue.

Even towards the close of the colonial era, the Bhore Committee, for all its criticism of existing public services and its emphatic support for better health care for women, remained cautious and divided on the issue. It is one of the many paradoxes of late colonial India that, while the issue of 'population' featured prominently in official discourse from the 1870s onwards and powerfully articulated ideas of an India that was lamentably 'premodern' and enduringly subjected to 'Nature', the state was unable to identify itself openly and wholeheartedly, either in discourse or in practice, with the kinds of medical and public health measures that might have done most to accelerate the advent of that modernity—including measures relating to women's health.

It may be asked whether the growth of a class of women trained in biomedicine had any significant impact on women's health care. It cannot be denied that the growth of a class of women doctors trained in biomedicine meant that an occupational identity was created for them, which laid the foundation for the development of a class of women practitioners in future. No doubt, the issues of power, hierarchy, and stratification within the medical profession along axes of gender, race, class, and community played a dominant role in somewhat limiting the significance of the growth of medical education for women. Indian women doctors trained in biomedicine had to struggle hard to find suitable jobs within governmental and Dufferin hospitals. Women belonging to the middle classes also faced resentment of family members in case of their interaction with lower castes and, in some cases, Muslim clients.[12]

Fortunate women patients were offered more options of choosing from different kinds of practitioners, including qualified male and female practitioners of Western medicine as well as those of indigenous medicine. Among members of the WMS, there was a clear commitment to investigating and improving reproductive health. In the late colonial period, there appeared to have been no consensus about the desirability of propagating birth control and what was done received little publicity. It, however, must be remembered that the practitioners of biomedicine did not singularly dominate the health care system in India. Yashoda Devi of Allahabad was a famous ayurvedic practitioner at the beginning of the twentieth century. She wrote more than forty books on the different aspects of women's health.[13] Ayurvedic practitioner Vimla Devi Vaidya wrote a pamphlet titled *Garbh Nirodh* in 1940, where she discussed available methods of birth control, drawing selectively from biomedicine as well as from traditional methods. Practitioners of both biomedicine and indigenous medicine in India saw birth control as a useful device for extending their elitist agenda of surveillance and exerting power over the lives of the working classes and other subaltern groups. However, unlike many, Vimla Devi argued that the working classes had low fertility rates. She advocated disciplining of sexual habits for the growth of strong, healthy, masculine bodies as the ideals for national bodies.[14]

In case of birth control, indigenous practitioners wrote in favour of both the new biomedical as well as the more traditional methods of birth control. Although practitioners of biomedicine and of alternative traditions of medicine in colonial India were divided among themselves on the issue of birth control, it appears that they 'shared a common agenda of marginalizing practising midwives and discrediting their hold on the bodies of Indian women.'[15] It would be fair to conclude that all medical participants in discussions on contraception in colonial India—foreign advocates, Indian middle-class men and women proponents, biomedical practitioners, and practitioners of alternative medicine—articulated the issue of birth control as one of surveillance and restraint. Birth control became a site for regulating and disciplining subaltern bodies, feeding into the elite hegemonic projects of neo-Malthusianism, eugenics, nationalism, and even feminism. Those biomedical physicians and indigenous practitioners who supported birth control voiced their support for ideas of regulation and discipline rather than seeking to empower their patients.

Medical journals document the many instances when Indian women refused to comply with the biomedical injunctions on birthing and the sway of dhais. Sanjam Ahluwalia's interviews of Jaunpuri dhais bring out very clearly the subaltern perspectives that are absent in the elite narratives of medical practitioners. These dhais held a high place of honour within the local community. They not only provided skilled services during childbirth but also helped in solving other gynaecological problems. Sometimes elite narratives also carry within themselves registration of resistance to their oppressive agendas. Correlating data from biomedical journals and oral interviews like those taken in Kanpur, it becomes clear that hegemonic assertions and medical interventions might attempt to shape the contours of modernist normative discourse and practice of health and otherize local knowledge, but cannot claim homogeneity and mono-cultural dominance.[16] In post-1947 India, 'population explosion' is often blamed as one of the leading challenges to the country's development and fertility control is advocated as one of the means of solving India's problems. Evidently, the construction of demographic factor and contraceptive usage as the markers of national progress do not reflect any break from the past. So also, there are deep-rooted historical links behind features like differential access to health care between men and women because of cultural and societal factors, high concentration of health care system in urban areas, high rates of maternal mortality compared to most emerging economies, and low percentage of women health workers in rural areas, which adversely affect women's health in India today. It may not be irrelevant to point out in this connection that in recent years a wish to break away from past approaches has become visible. Several non-governmental organizations, researchers, and women's groups in India have raised the issue of moving away from demographic goals to address the needs of clients (especially women). It may not be wrong to suggest that a paradigmatic shift is noticeable in different discussions, which tends to highlight the need for adding intervention in sexually transmitted diseases, HIV, and AIDS in the agenda of family planning and reproductive health organizations in recent years. A full and detailed discussion on these aspects, however, lies outside the scope of this work.[17]

Notes and References

1. *Report of the Health Survey and Development Committee* 1 (Delhi: Manager of Publications, 1946), p. 9; David Arnold, 'Official Attitudes to Population, Birth Control and Reproductive Health in India, 1921–1946', in *Reproductive Health in India: History, Politics, Controversies*, edited by Sara Hodges (New Delhi: Orient Longman, 2006), p. 45.

2. Allan Webb, *Pathologica Indica, or, the Anatomy of Indian Diseases, Medical and Surgical: Based upon Morbid Specimens from All Parts of India in the Museum of the Calcutta Medical College; Illustrated by Detailed Cases, with the Prescriptions and Treatment Employed, and Comments, Physiological, Practical and Historical*, 2nd edition (London: W.H. Allen and Co., 1848), pp. 254–60. Also cited in Ishita Pande, *Medicine, Race and Liberalism in British Bengal: Symptoms of Empire* (London and New York: Routledge, 2010), p. 155.

3. John Roberton, *Essays and Notes on the Physiology and Diseases of Women, and on Practical Midwifery* (London: John Churchill, 1851). Also cited in Pande, *Medicine, Race and Liberalism in British Bengal*, pp. 153–4.

4. Roberton, *Essays and Notes on the Physiology and Diseases of Women*, p. 22. Also cited in Pande, *Medicine, Race and Liberalism in British Bengal*, p. 154.

5. Pande, *Medicine, Race and Liberalism in British Bengal*, p. 225.

6. Fever Hospital Committee, *Abridgement of the Report of the Committee Appointed by the Right Honorable the Governor of Bengal for the Establishment of a Fever Hospital and for Inquiring into Local Management and Taxation in Calcutta* (Calcutta: 1840).

7. Fever Hospital Committee, *Abridgement of the Report of the Committee*, p. 64. Cited in Pande, *Medicine, Race and Liberalism in British Bengal*, p. 144.

8. Sumanta Banerjee, 'Marginalization of Women's Popular Culture in Nineteenth Century Bengal', in *Recasting Women: Essays in Colonial History*, edited by Kumkum Sangari and Suresh Vaid (New Delhi: Kali for Women, 1989).

9. Pande, *Medicine, Race and Liberalism in British Bengal*, p. 147.

10. Pande, *Medicine, Race and Liberalism in British Bengal*, p. 147.

11. Pande, *Medicine, Race and Liberalism in British Bengal*, p. 147.

12. See Sanjam Ahluwalia, *Reproductive Restraints: Birth Control in India 1877–1947* (New Delhi: Permanent Black, 2008), p. 165.

13. See Charu Gupta, *Sexuality, Obscenity, Community: Women, Muslims and the Hindu Public in Colonial India* (New Delhi: Permanent Black, 2001), pp. 185–90.

14. Ahluwalia, *Reproductive Restraints*, pp. 165–72.

15. Ahluwalia, *Reproductive Restraints*, pp. 184–5.

16. Ahluwalia, *Reproductive Restraints*, pp. 184–5.

17. Ashish Bose, 'The Family Welfare Programme in India: Changing Paradigm' in *The Family Welfare Programme in India,* edited by H.M. Mathur (New Delhi: Vikas Publishing, 1995), pp. 1–29. S. Pachauri, ed., *Implementing a Reproductive Health Agenda in India: The Beginning* (New Delhi: Population Council Regional Office, 1999); *Integrating STI Management into family Planning Services: What Are the Benefits,* WHO Occasional Paper, no. 1, pub. order no. WHO/RHR/99.10 (World Health Organization: Geneva, Switzerland, 1999).

Bibliography

Primary Sources

National Archives of India, New Delhi.

Government of India, Files and Proceedings.

Home Proceedings, 1888–1933.

Education, Establishment, Jails, Judicial, Medical, Police, Public, Sanitary Branches.

West Bengal State Archives, Calcutta.

Proceedings of the Government of Bengal: 1835 to 1945–6, General (Miscellaneous) Branch, Public Health Branch, Education Branch, Medical Branch, Municipal Branch, Sanitary Branch.

Proceedings of Local Self-Government Department, Agriculture and Industries Department.

Private Papers

All India Women's Conference (AIWC) Papers, Kamaladevi Chattopadhyaya Papers. Nehru Memorial Museum and Library, New Delhi.

Manilal, B. *Nanavati Papers: Memoranda and Oral Proceedings of the Famine Commission, 1944–1945*. National Archives of India, New Delhi.

Newspapers and Periodicals

English

Amrita Bazar Patrika
Bengalee
Brahmo Public Opinion
Calcutta Review
Englishwoman's Review
Forward
Hindoo Patriot
Indian Journal of Medical Research
Indian Medical Gazette
Indian Mirror
Journal of the Association of Medical Women in India
Journal of the Indian Medical Association
Lancet
Modern Review
Calcutta Medical Journal 19, no. 3 (1924)
Statesman

Bengali

Antahpur
Bamabodhini Patrika
Banga Lakshmi
Bharati
Bharat Mahila
Chikitsa Sammilani
Dainik Basumati
Desh
Mahila
Probasi
Swasthya
Vigyan Darpan

Other Official Reports and Publications

Age of Consent Committee Evidence, volumes 1–9. Calcutta: Government Publications, 1929.

All India Institute of Hygiene and Public Health, *Annual Reports*.

An Appeal on Behalf of the Calcutta School of Tropical Medicine and Hygiene and the Carmichael Hospital for Tropical Diseases. Calcutta: Bengal Secretariat Press, 1920.

Annual and Triennial Reports on the Working of Hospitals and Dispensaries in Bengal by Surgeon-General with the Government of Bengal.

Annual and Triennial Reports on Vaccination in Bengal, Bengal Public Health Department.

Annual Report of the Medical Schools in Bengal: 1914–1919.

Annual Reports of the All India Institute of Hygiene and Public Health, Calcutta.

Annual Reports of the Bengal Branch of the Countess of Dufferin Fund. Annual Reports of the Director of Public Health for Bengal.

Annual Reports of the National Association for Supplying Medical Aid by Women to Women in India (Dufferin Fund).

Annual Reports of the Public Health Commissioner with the Government of India.

Annual Reports of the Saroj Nalini Dutta Memorial Association, from the year 1925 to 1931, Calcutta.

Annual Reports of the Tuberculosis Association of Bengal.

Annual Reports of the Tuberculosis Association of India.

Bengal Legislative Council and Assembly Proceedings.

Bengal Public Health Reports, Public Health Department, Government of Bengal.

Census of India, Bengal, 1881, 1891, 1901,1911,1921,1931.

Census of India, Calcutta, Towns and Suburbs, 1891, 1901,1911,1921,1931.

Centenary Volume of Calcutta Medical College, Calcutta, 1935.

Central Advisory Board of Health (CABH). *Report on Maternity and Child Welfare Work in India by Special Committee (1938)*. Simla: Manager, Government of India Press, 1939.

'Discussion on Organisation of Child Welfare Work'. *Proceedings of the Seventh Congress of the Far Eastern Association for Tropical Medicine, Calcutta, December 1927*. Calcutta: Government of India Press, 1928.

Famine Inquiry Commission. *Final Report, 1945*. Delhi: Manager of Publications, 1945.

Famine Inquiry Commission. *Report on Bengal, by* Sir John Woodhead. Delhi: Manager of Publications, 1945.

Fever Hospital Committee. *Abridgement of the Report of the Committee Appointed by the Right Honorable the Governor of Bengal for the Establishment of a Fever Hospital and for Inquiring into Local Management and Taxation in Calcutta.* Calcutta: 1840.

General Committee of Public Instruction. *Copybook of Letters.*

General Report on the Lunatic Asylums, Vaccination, and Dispensaries in the Bengal Presidency.

Government of Bengal. *Report on the Charitable Dispensaries.*

Health Bulletin 15: Maternal Mortality in Childbirth in India: A Summary of the Investigation Conducted under the Indian Research Fund Association 1925. Calcutta: 1928.

Native Female Medical Education in Bengal, the N.W. Provinces and Oudh and the Punjab, Home-Medical, 76/83, December, 1887. National Archives of India, New Delhi.

Printed Proceedings of the Governors of Native Hospital Dated 20th May 1835, with Notes and Proceedings of the General Committee from 18th June 1835 to 12th November 1840 (bound manuscript volume). [Also known as the Fever Hospital Committee Report.] West Bengal State Archives.

Proceedings of All India Medical Conference. Delhi: 1934.

Proceedings of the First All India Sanitary Conference Held at Bombay on 13th and 14th November 1911. Calcutta: Superintendent of Government Printing.

Proceedings of the General Malaria Committee. Simla: 1911–4.

Proceedings of the Sanitary Commission for Bengal. Calcutta: 1864–70.

Proceedings of the Second All India Sanitary Conference Held at Madras, November 11th to 16th, 1912, 1913. Simla: Government Central Branch Press, 1912.

Proceedings of the Seventh Congress of the Far Eastern Association for Tropical Medicine, Calcutta, December 1927. Calcutta: Government of India Press, 1928.

Report by Civil Medical Officers on the Nature, Growth and Mode of Preparation of the Various Alimentary Articles Consumed as Food by the Industrial and Labouring Population in the Several Districts of Bengal, North Western Provinces, Punjab, Oudh and British Burma. Calcutta: Home Secretariat Press, 1863.

Report of the Committee Appointed by Government to Observe and Report upon Surgical Operations by Dr. J. Esdaile upon Patients under the Influence of Alleged Mesmeric Agency, 1846. Calcutta: Military Orphan Press, 1846.

Report of the Committee for the Establishment of a Fever Hospital and for Inquiring into Local Management and Taxation in Calcutta. Calcutta: Bishop's College Press, 1840.

Report of the Committee on Prison Discipline, 1838. Calcutta: Baptist Mission Press.

Report of the Epidemics of Plague in Calcutta during the Years 1898–99, 1899–1900 up to 30th June 1900. Calcutta: Municipal Press, 1900.

Report of the Health Survey and Development Committee under Chairmanship of Sir Joseph Bhore. Delhi: Government of India Press, 1946.

Report of the Royal Commission on Agriculture, 1926–28.

Report of the Small Pox Commissioners. Calcutta: Military Orphan Press, 1850.

Report on the Cholera Epidemic of 1867 in Northern India. Calcutta: 1867.

Reports of the Calcutta Improvement Trust. Calcutta: 1911–14.

Reports of the Calcutta Medical Institutions, for different years.

Reports of the Commissioners for the Improvement of Calcutta. Calcutta: 1848–53.

Reports of the Indian Plague Commission, 5 vols. London: 1900.

Reports of the Municipal Administration of Calcutta, 1920–21.

Reports of the Sanitary Commissioner for the Government of Bengal. Calcutta: 1868–1915.

Reports of the Sanitary Commissioner with the Government of India. Calcutta: 1868–1915.

Reports on the Charitable Dispensaries of Bengal. Calcutta: 1869–1908.

Reports on the Working of District Boards in Bengal. Calcutta: 1889–1915.

Reports on the Working of Municipality in Bengal. Calcutta: 1889–1915.

Reports on Vaccination in the Province of Bengal. Calcutta: 1867–81.

Sanitary Commissioner (Bengal). *Investigations on Bengal Jail Dietaries with Some Observations on the Influence of the Dietary on the Physical Development and Well-being of the People of Bengal*. Calcutta: Superintendent of Government Printing, 1910.

The Countess of Dufferin's Fund—the Sixth Annual Report of the National Association for Supplying Female Medical Aid to the Women of India, Burma Branch, for the Year 1892. Calcutta: Office of the Superintendent of Government Printing, 1893.

Transactions of all the All India Sanitary Conferences. Calcutta: 1911–14.

Secondary

Books

Ackerknecht, Erwin H. *Medicine at the Paris Hospital: 1794–1848*. Baltimore: The Johns Hopkins University Press, 1967.

Adas, Michael. 'Scientific Standards and Colonial Education in British India and French Senegal'. In *Science, Medicine and Cultural Imperialism*, edited by Teresa Meade and Mark Walker, 4–35. Basingstoke: Macmillan, 1991.

Ahluwalia, Sanjam. 'Controlling Births, Policing Sexualities: A History of Birth Control in Colonial India, 1877–1946.' PhD diss., University of Cincinnati, 2000.

———. *Reproductive Restraints: Birth Control in India 1877–1947*. New Delhi: Permanent Black, 2008.

Alavi, Seema. *Islam and Healing: Loss and Recovery of an Indo-Muslim Medical Tradition*. Basingstoke: Palgrave Macmillan, 2008.

Amin, Sonia Nishat. *The World of Muslim Women in Colonial Bengal: 1876–1939*. Leiden: Brill, 1996.

Anandhi, S. 'Reproductive Bodies and Regulated Sexuality: Birth Control Debates in Early Twentieth Century Tamilnadu.' In *A Question of Silence? The Sexual Economies of Modern India*, edited by Mary E. John and Janaki Nair, 139–66. Delhi: Kali for Women, 1998.

Anderson, Benedict. *Imagined Communities: Reflections on the Origin and Spread of Nationalism*, revised and extended edition. London: Verso, 1991.

Anderson, Warwick. 'Immunities of Empire: Race, Disease, and the New Tropical Medicine.' *Bulletin of the History of Medicine* 70, no. 1 (1996): 94–118.

Annesley, James. *Researches into the Causes, Nature and Treatment of the Most Prevalent Diseases of India and of Warm Climates Generally*, 2 vols. London: Longman, Rees, Orme, Brown and Green, 1828.

Anonymous. 'The Problem of Midwifery Training in Indian Medical Colleges.' *Calcutta Medical Journal* 19, no. 3 (1924): 158–60.

Appadurai, Arjun. *Modernity at Large: Cultural Dimensions of Globalization*. Minneapolis: University of Minnesota Press, 1996.

Armstrong, David. 'Bodies of Knowledge/Knowledge of Bodies.' In *Reassessing Foucault: Power, Medicine and the Body*, edited by Colin Jones and Roy Porter. London and New York: Routledge, 1995.

Arnold, David. *Colonizing the Body: State Medicine and Epidemic Disease in Nineteenth-Century India*. Berkeley, California: University of California Press, 1993.

———. 'The "Discovery" of Malnutrition and Diet in Colonial India.' *Indian Economic and Social History Review* 31, no. 1 (1994): 1–26.

———. 'Official Attitudes to Population, Birth Control and Reproductive Health in India, 1921–1946.' In Hodges, *Reproductive Health in India*, 22–50.

———. *Science, Technology and Medicine in Colonial India*. Vol. 3, part 5 of *The New Cambridge History of India*. Cambridge: Cambridge University Press, 2000.

———. 'Sexually Transmitted Diseases in Nineteenth- and Twentieth-Century India.' *Genitourinary Medicine* 69 (February 1993): 3–8.

Arnold, David. 'Social Crisis and Epidemic Disease in the Famines of Nineteenth Century India'. *Social History of Medicine* 6, no. 3 (1993): 385–404.

———. *The Tropics and the Traveling Gaze: India, Landscape, and Science, 1800–1856*. Seattle: University of Washington Press, 2006.

———, ed. *Warm Climates and Western Medicine: The Emergence of Tropical Medicine, 1500–1900*. Volume 35 of *Clio Medica S./Wellcome Institute Series in the History of Medicine* Series. Amsterdam: Rodopi, 1996.

Attewell, Guy N.A. *Refiguring Unani Tibb: Plural Healing in Late Colonial India*. New Delhi: Orient BlackSwan, 2007.

Baber, Zaheer. *The Science of Empire: Scientific Knowledge, Civilization, and Colonial Rule in India*. New Delhi: Oxford University Press, 1998.

Bagal, Jogesh C. 'History of Bethune School and College: 1849–1949'. In Nag, *Bethune School & College Centenary Volume*.

Bagchi, Amiya Kumar and Krishna Soman, eds. *Maladies, Preventives and Curatives: Debates in Public Health in India*. New Delhi: Tulika Books, 2005.

Bagchi, Jasodhara. 'Representing Nationalism: Ideology of Motherhood in Colonial Bengal'. *Economic and Political Weekly* 25, no. 42/43 (1990): WS65–WS71.

Bala, Poonam. *Imperialism and Medicine in Bengal: A Socio-Historical Perspective*. New Delhi: SAGE Publications, 1991.

Balfour, John. *A Sexual Science: A Guidebook for Married and Single Men*. Bombay: Century Publishing Co., 1894.

Balfour, Margaret. 'Maternal Mortality in Childbirth in India'. *JAMWI* 16, no. 1 (1928): 5–25.

Balfour, Margaret I. and Ruth Young. *The Work of Medical Women in India*. London: Oxford University Press, 1929.

Ballhatchet, Kenneth. *Race, Sex and Class under the Raj: Imperial Attitudes and Policies and Their Critics, 1793–1905*. London: Weidenfeld and Nicolson, 1980.

Ballingall, George. *Outlines of the Course of Lectures on Military Surgery, Delivered in the University of Edinburgh*. Edinburgh: Adam Black, 1833.

Bandopadhyaya, Arun. *Science and Society in India, C. 1750–2000*. New Delhi: Manohar, 2010.

Bandyopadhyay, Brajendranath. *Dwarakanath Gangopadhyay*. Calcutta: Bangiya Sahitya Parishad, 1952.

Bandyopadhyay, Sekhar, ed. *Bengal: Rethinking History: Essays in Historiography*. New Delhi: Manohar, 2001.

———. *From Plassey to Partition: A History of Modern India*. New Delhi: Orient Longman, 2004.

Bandyopadhyay, Tarasankar. *Arogyaniketan*. Translated into English by Enakshi Chatterjee. New Delhi: Sahitya Academy, 1996.

Banerjee, Madhulika. *Power, Knowledge, Medicine: Ayurvedic Pharmaceuticals at Home and in the World*. Hyderabad: Orient BlackSwan, 2009.

Banerjee, Sumanta. 'The "Beshya" and the "Babu": The Prostitute and Her Clientele in Nineteenth-Century Bengal'., *Economic and Political Weekly* 28, no. 45 (1993): 2461–72.

———. 'Marginalization of Women's Popular Culture in Nineteenth Century Bengal'. In Sangari and Vaid, *Recasting Women*, 127–79.

Bannerji, Himani. 'Fashioning a Self: Educational Proposals for and by Women in Popular Magazines in Colonial Bengal'. *Economic and Political Weekly* 26, no. 43 (1991).

———. *Inventing Subjects: Studies in Hegemony, Patriarchy, and Colonialism*. London: Anthem Press, 2002.

Bartley, Paula. *Prostitution: Prevention and Reform in England, 1860–1914*. New York: Routledge, 2000.

Basu, Aparna. 'A Century and a Half's Journey: Women's Education in India, 1850s to 2000'. In *Women of India: Colonial and Post-Colonial Periods*, edited by Bharati Ray, 183–207. New Delhi/Thousand Oaks/London: SAGE Publications, 2005.

———. *The Growth of Education and Political Development in India: 1898–1920*. New Delhi: Oxford University Press, 1974.

———. 'The Indian Response to Scientific and Technical Education in the Colonial Era, 1820–1920'. In D. Kumar, *Science and Empire*, pp. 126–38.

———. 'Mary Ann Cooke to Mother Teresa: Christian Missionary Women and Indian Response'. In *Women Missions: Past and Present: Anthropological and Historical Perceptions (Cross-Cultural Perspectives on Women)*, edited by Fiona Bowie, Deborah Kirkwood, and Shirley Ardener. Oxford: Berg, 1993.

Basu, Aparna and Bharati Ray. *Women's Struggle*. New Delhi: Manohar, 1990.

Basu, Raj Sekhar. 'Medical Missionaries at Work: The Canadian Baptist Missionaries in a Native Indian State: The Case of the LMS in Travancore, 1866–1950'. Kumar, *Disease and Medicine in India*, pp. 180–97.

Batabyal, Rakesh. *Communalism in Bengal: From Famine to Noakhali, 1943–47*. SAGE Series in Modern Indian History VI. New Delhi: SAGE Publications, 2005.

Bayly, C.A. *Empire and Information: Intelligence Gathering and Social Communication in India, 1780–1870*. Cambridge: Cambridge University Press, 1996.

Beilby, E. 'Medical Women for India'. *Journal of the National Indian Association* 176 (1885): 357–65.

Bentley, C.A. *Report of an Investigation into the Causes of Malaria in Bombay and the Measures Necessary for Its Control*. Bombay: Government Central Press, 1911.

Bhabha, Homi K. *The Location of Culture*. London: Routledge, 1994.

———, ed. *Nation and Narration*. London: Routledge, 1990.

Bhatia, B.M. *Famines in India: A Study in Some Aspects of the Economic History of India, 1860–1965*, 2nd edition. Bombay: Asia Publishing House, 1967.

Bhattacharya, Jayanta. 'Anatomical Knowledge and East–West Exchange'. In *Medical Encounters in British India*, edited by Deepak Kumar and Raj Sekhar Basu, 40–60. New Delhi: Oxford University Press, 2013.

———. 'The Genesis of Hospital Medicine in India: The Calcutta Medical College (CMC) and the Emergence of a New Medical Epistemology'. *Indian Economic and Social History Review* 51 (2014): 231–64.

Bhattacharya, Sanjay. *Expunging Variola: The Control and Eradication of Small Pox in India, 1947–77*. Hyderabad: Orient Longman, 2006.

Bhattacharya, Sanjay, Mark Harrison, and Michael Worboys. *Fractured States: Small Pox, Public Health and Vaccination Policy in British India, 1800–1947*. Hyderabad: Orient Longman, 2005.

Bhattacharya, Tithi. *The Sentinels of Culture: Class, Education, and the Colonial Intellectuals in Bengal*. New Delhi: Oxford University Press, 2005.

Billington, Mary Frances. *Women in India*. London: Chapman and Hall, 1895.

Biswas, Arun Kumar. *Collected Works of Mahendralal Sircar, Eugene Lafont and the Science Movement (1860–1910)*. Kolkata: Asiatic Society, 2001.

Blake, Catriona. *The Charge of the Parasols: Women's Entry to the Medical Profession*. London: The Women's Press, 1990.

Borthwick, Meredith. *The Changing Role of Women in Bengal, 1849–1905*. Princeton: Princeton University Press, 1984.

———. *Keshub Chunder Sen: A Search for Cultural Synthesis*. Calcutta: Minerva Associates, 1977.

Bose, Ashish. 'The Family Welfare Programme in India: Changing Paradigm'. In *The Family Welfare Programme in India*, edited by H.M. Mathur, 1–29. New Delhi: Vikas Publishing, 1995.

Bose, Chunilal. 'Diet of the Bengalis'. In his, *Food: The Adharchandra Mookerjee Lectures for 1929*, 92–110. Calcutta: University of Calcutta, 1930.

Bose, Pradip Kumar, ed. *Health and Society in Bengal: A Selection from Late 19th-Century Bengali Periodicals*. New Delhi/Thousand Oaks/London: SAGE Publications, 2006.

———. 'Sons of the Nation: Child Rearing in the New Family'. In *Texts of Power: Emerging Disciplines in Colonial Bengal*, edited by Partha Chatterjee. Calcutta: Samya, 1996.

Bose, Rajnarain. *Se Kal ar E Kal*. Calcutta: 1976 [1874].

Bose, S.C. *The Hindoos as They Are: A Description of the Manners, Customs and Inner Life of Hindoo Society in Bengal*. Calcutta: 1881.

Bose, Sugata. *Agrarian Bengal: Economy, Social Structure and Politics, 1919–47*. Cambridge: Cambridge University Press, 1986.

Briggs, Laura. *Reproducing Empire: Race, Sex, Science, and U.S. Imperialism in Puerto Rico*. California: University of California Press, 2002.

Burton, Antoinette. *Burdens of History: British Feminists, Indian Women and Imperial Culture, 1865–1915*. Chapel Hill, London: University of North Carolina, 1994.

———. 'From Child Bride to "Hindoo Lady": Rukhmabai and the Debate on Sexual Respectability in Imperial Britain'. *American Historical Review* 103, no. 4 (1998): 1119–46.

———. 'Contesting the Zenana: The Mission to Make "Lady Doctors for India", 1874–1885'. *Journal of British Studies* 35, no. 3 (1996): 368–97.

———. *Dwelling in the Archive: Women Writing House, Home, and History in Late Colonial India*. New York: Oxford University Press, 2003.

———. 'The White Woman's Burden: British Feminists and the "Indian Woman", 1865–1915'. In N. Choudhuri and Strobel, *Western Women and Imperialism*, pp. 137–57.

Bynum, W.F. 'Malaria in Inter-War British India'. *Parasitologia* 42 (2000): 25–31.

Chakrabarti, Pratik. 'Medical Marketplace beyond the West: Bazaar Medicine, Trade and the English Establishment in Eighteenth Century India'. In *Medicine and the Market in Early Modern England and Its Colonies*, edited by Patrick Wallis and Mark Jenner, 196–215. Basingstoke: Palgrave Macmillan, 2007.

———. *Western Science in Modern India: Metropolitan Methods, Colonial Practices*. New Delhi: Permanent Black, 2004.

Chakrabarty, Dipesh. 'The Difference-Deferral of (A) Colonial Modernity: Public Debates on Domesticity in British Bengal'. *History Workshop* 36, no. 1 (1993): 1–34.

———. *Habitations of Modernity: Essays in the Wake of Subaltern Studies*. Chicago: University of Chicago Press, 2002.

———. 'Open Space/Public Place: Garbage, Modernity and India', *South Asia* 14, no. 1 (1991): 15–31.

———. 'Postcoloniality and the Artifice of History'. In *A Subaltern Studies Reader: 1986–1995*, edited by Ranajit Guha. Minneapolis: University of Minnesota Press, 1997.

———. *Provincializing Europe: Postcolonial Thought and Historical Difference*. Princeton, New Jersey: Princeton University Press, 2000.

Chakraborty, Usha. *Conditions of Bengali Women around the 2nd Half of the 19th Century*. Calcutta: Self-published, 1963.

Chakravarty, Renu. *Communists in Indian Women's Movement, 1940–50*. New Delhi: Peoples' Publishing House, 1980.

Chakravarty, Uma. 'Whatever Happened to the Vedic Dasi?' in Sangari and Vaid, *Recasting Women*, pp. 27–87.

Chandravarkar, Rajnarayan. 'Plague Panic and Epidemic Politics in India: 1896–1914'. In *Epidemics and Ideas: Essays on the Historical Perception of Pestilence*, edited by Terence O. Ranger and Paul Slack, 203–40. Cambridge: Cambridge University Press, 1999.

Chatterjee, Partha. *Bengal, 1920–47: The Land Question*. Calcutta: K.P. Bagchi & Co., 1984.

———. *The Nation and Its Fragments: Colonial and Postcolonial Histories*. New Delhi: Oxford University Press, 1992.

———. 'The Nationalist Resolution of the Women's Question'. In Sangari and Vaid, *Recasting Women*, pp. 233–53.

———. *Nationalist Thought and the Colonial World: A Derivative Discourse*. New Delhi: Oxford University Press, 1986.

Chatterjee, Ratnabali. 'The Indian Prostitute as a Colonial Subject, Bengal 1864–1883'. *Canadian Woman Studies/Les Cahiers de la Femme* 13, no. 1 (1992): 51–5.

Chatterjee, Srilata. 'Colonial Women, Medicine and Medical Education in Bengal 1884–1940'. In *Women's Education and Politics of Gender*, edited by Uttara Chakraborty and Banimanjari Das, 103–23. 125 year commemoration volume. Calcutta: Bethune College, 2004.

Chattopadhyay, Debiprasad. *Science and Society in Ancient India*. Kolkata: Research India Publications, 1977.

Chattopadhyay, Swati. *Representing Calcutta: Modernity, Nationalism and the Colonial Uncanny*. London: Routledge, 2006.

Chaudhuri, B.B. 'Agrarian Economy and Agrarian Relations in Bengal, 1859–85'. In Sinha, *History of Bengal*.

———. 'Agricultural Production in Bengal: Coexistence of Decline and Growth, 1859–1885'. *Bengal Past and Present* 88, part 2, no. 166 (1969).

———. 'Growth of Commercial Agriculture in Bengal, 1859–1885'. *Indian Economic and Social History Review* 7 (1970): 25–60.

———. 'The Process of Depeasantisation in Bengal and Bihar, 1885–1947'. *Indian Historical Review* 21, no. 1 (1975): 105–65.

Chaudhuri, Nupur and Margaret Strobel, eds. *Western Women and Imperialism: Complicity and Resistance*. Bloomington: Indiana University Press, 1992.

Chaudhuri, Tripti. 'Women in Radical Movements in Bengal in the 1940s: The Story of the Mahila Atmaraksha Samiti (Women's Self-Defence League)'. In *Faces of the Feminine in Ancient, Medieval and Modern India*, edited by Mandakranta Bose. New Delhi: Oxford University Press, 2000.

Chevers, Norman. *A Commentary on the Disease of India*. London: Churchill, 1886.

Choudhary, B.K. *Tuberculosis in India: A Political Ecology Approach*. Saarbruecken: VDM Verlag, 2008.

Chowdhury, Indira. *Frail Hero and Virile History: Gender and the Politics of Culture in Colonial Bengal*. New Delhi: Oxford University Press, 1998.

Clark, John. *Observations on the Diseases in Long Voyages to Hot Countries and Particularly on Those Which Prevail in the East Indies*. London: Wilson and Nicol, 1773.

———. 'Report on Syphilis in H.M. Light Dragoons'. *Madras Quarterly Medical Journal* 1 (1839): 370–410.

Cohn, Bernard S. *Colonialism and Its Forms of Knowledge: The British in India*. New Delhi: Oxford University Press, 1999.

Collingham, Elizabeth M. *Imperial Bodies: The Physical Experience of the Raj, C. 1800–1947*. Cambridge: Polity Press, 2001.

Comaroff, Jean and John L. Comaroff. 'Home-Made Hegemony: Modernity, Domesticity, and Colonialism in South Africa'. In *African Encounters with Domesticity*, edited by K. Hansen. New Brunswick: Rutgers University Press, 1992.

Crawford, D.G. *Role of the Indian Medical Service: 1615*–1930. London: Thacker & Co., 1930.

Crosby, Alfred W. *Ecological Imperialism: The Biological Expansion of Europe 900–1900*. Cambridge: Cambridge University Press, 1986.

Cunningham, A. and B. Andrew, eds. *Western Medicine as Contested Knowledge*. Manchester: Manchester University Press, 1997.

Curjel, D. *Improvement of the Conditions of Childbirth in India*. Calcutta: Bengal Secretariat Book Depot, 1918.

Curtin, Philip D. *Death by Migration: Europe's Encounter with the Tropical World in the Nineteenth Century*. Cambridge: Cambridge University Press, 1989.

———. *The Image of Africa: British Ideas and Action, 1780–1850*. Madison: University of Wisconsin Press, 1964.

Dandeker, Christopher. *Surveillance, Power, and Modernity: Bureaucracy and Discipline from 1700 to the Present Day*. New York: St Martin's Press, 1990.

Das, Amal. 'Calcutta Plague: Epidemic, Colonial Intervention and Indigenous Society, 1898–1900'. In Palit and Dutta, *History of Medicine in India*, pp. 87–110.

Das, Anirban. 'Medical Knowledge of the Body: Colonial Encounters'. *Re-thinking Marxism* 13, no. 2 (2001): 109–31.

Das, Debjani. *Houses of Madness: Insanity and Asylums of Bengal in Nineteenth-Century India*. New Delhi: Oxford University Press, 2015.

Das, Tarak Chandra. *Bengal Famine (1943), As Revealed in a Survey of the Destitute in Calcutta*. Calcutta: University of Calcutta, 1949.

Das Gupta, Sanjukta. *Adivasis and the Raj: Socio-Economic Transition of the Hos, 1820–1932*. New Delhi: Orient BlackSwan, 2011.

Datta, Haridhan. *Narijibane Dehatattva o Svasthya Vishayak Sadharaner Pathyopayogi Pustak*. Calcutta: Chakrabarti & Co., 1906.

Datta, Partho. 'Ranald Martin's *Medical Topography* (1837): The Emergence of Public Health in Calcutta'. In *The Social History of Health and Medicine in Colonial India*, edited by Biswamoy Pati and Mark Harrison, 15–30. London and New York: Routledge, 2009.

Davidoff, Leonore and Catherine Hall. *Family Fortunes: Men and Women of the English Middle Class, 1780–1850*. Chicago: University of Chicago Press, 1987.

Davin, Anna. 'Imperialism and Motherhood'. *History Workshop Journal* 5 (1978): 9–66.

Day, Lal Behari. *Bengal Peasant Life*. London: Macmillan & Co. Limited, 1913.

Deb, Radha Kanta. 'Account of the Thikadars'. *Transactions of the Medical and Physical Society of Calcutta* 5 (1831): 416–18.

Deb, Shib Chunder. *Sisupalan*, part I. Serampore: 1857; part 2. Calcutta: 1862.

Deb Roy, Rohan. '"An Awful, Unseen Visitant": The Return of Burdwan Fever'. *Economic and Political Weekly* 43, nos 12–13 (2008): 62–70.

DeBary, W.T. *Sources of Indian Tradition*. New York: Columbia University Press, 1968.

Dey, Kanny Lal. *Hindu Social Laws and Habits Viewed in Relation to Health*. Kolkata: R.C. Lepage,1866.

Dutta, Gurusaday. *Woman of India, Being the Life of Saroj Nalini*. London: Weidenfield and Nicholson, 1929.

Dutta, Prankrishna, *Kolikatar Itibritto o Onyanyo Rachana*, edited by Debasis Bose. Calcutta: Pustak Bipani, 1991.

Dutta, Ramesh Chandra. *Indian Famines: Their Cause and Prevention*. London: P.S. King, 1901.

Dutta Gupta, Sarmistha. *Identities and Histories: Women's Writings and Politics in Bengal*. Kolkata: Stree, 1999.

Dyson, T., ed. *India's Historical Demography: Studies in Famine, Disease and Society*. London: Curzon Press Limited, 1989.

Engels, Dagmar. *Beyond Purdah? Women in Bengal: 1890–1939*. New Delhi: Oxford University Press, 1996.

———. 'Modes of Knowledge, Modes of Power: Universities in Nineteenth-Century India'. In Engels and Marks, *Contesting Colonial Hegemony*, pp. 87–109.

Engels, Dagmar. 'The Politics of Childbirth: British and Bengali Women in Contest, 1890–1930'. In *Society and Ideology: Essays in South Asian History*, edited by Peter Robb, 222–46. New Delhi: Oxford University Press, 1993.

Engels, Dagmar and Shula Marks, eds. *Contesting Colonial Hegemony: State and Society in Africa and India*. London: British Academic Press, 1994.

Ernst, Waltraud. 'Beyond East and West: From the History of Colonial Medicine to a Social History of Medicine(s) in South Asia'. *Social History of Medicine* 20, no. 3 (2007): 505–24.

———. 'Colonial Psychiatry, Magic and Religion: The Case of Mesmerism in British India'. *History of Psychiatry* 15, no. 1 (2004): 57–71.

———. 'The Establishment of "Native Lunatic Asylums" in Early Nineteenth-Century British India'. In *Studies in Indian Medical History*, edited by G.J. Meulenbeld and D. Wujastyk, revised edition, 169–204. Delhi: Motilal Banarasidass, 2001.

———. 'European Madness and Gender in Nineteenth Century British India'. *Social History of Medicine* 9, no. 3 (1996): 357–82.

———. 'Feminising Madness—Feminising the Orient: Madness, Gender and Colonialism in British India, 1860–1040'. In Kak and Pati, *Exploring Gender Equations*, pp. 57–91.

———. 'Under the Influence in British India: Esdaile & the Critics of his "Mesmeric Hospital" in Calcutta'. *Psychological Medicine* 25 (1995): 1113–23.

———. *Mad Tales from the Raj: European Insane in British India*. London: Routledge, 1991.

———, ed. *Plural Medicine, Tradition and Modernity, 1800–2000*. London: Routledge, 2002.

Esdaile, J. *The Introduction of Mesmerism into the Public Hospitals of India*. London: W. Ken, 1856 [1852].

———. *Mesmerism in India and Its Practical Application in Surgery and Medicine*. London: Longman, 1846.

Fanon, Franz. 'Medicine and Colonialism'. In *The Cultural Crisis of Modern Medicine*, edited by J. Ehrenreich, 229–51. New York: Monthly Review Press, 1978.

Fielding, Michael, ed. *Birth Control in Asia: A Report of a Conference Held at the London School of Hygiene and Tropical Medicine, November 24–25 1933*. London: Birth Control International Information Centre, 1935.

Fitzgerald, Rosemary. '"Making and Moulding the Nursing of the Indian Empire": Recasting Nurses in Colonial India'. In Powell and Hurley, *Rhetoric and Reality*, pp. 185–222.

Forbes, Geraldine. 'Colonial Imperatives and Women's Emancipation: Western Medical Education for Indian Women in Nineteenth Century Bengal'. *Modern Historical Studies* 2 (2001): 83–102.

Forbes, Geraldine. 'The Issue of Child Marriage in India.' *Women's Studies International Quarterly* 2 (1979).

———. 'Managing Midwifery in India.' In Engels and Marks, *Contesting Colonial Hegemony: State and Society in Africa and India*, pp. 152–72.

———. 'Medical Careers and Health Care for Indian Women: Patterns of Control'. *Women's History Review* 3, no. 4 (1994): 515–30.

———. 'Negotiating Modernities: The Public and Private Worlds of Dr. Haimabati Sen.' In Powell and Lambert-Hurley, *Rhetoric and Reality*.

———. 'In Search of the "Pure Heathen": Missionary Women in Nineteenth-Century India.' *Economic and Political Weekly* 21 (1986): WS 2–8.

———. *Women in Colonial India: Essays on Politics, Medicine, and Historiography*. New Delhi: Chronicle Books, 2005.

———. *Women in Modern India*. Vol. 4, part 2 of *The New Cambridge History of India*. Cambridge: Cambridge University Press, first South Asian paperback edition, 1998.

Forbes, Geraldine and Tapan Raychaudhuri, eds. *The Memoirs of Dr. Haimabati Sen: From Child Widow to Lady Doctor*. New Delhi: Roli Books, 2000.

Foucault, Michel. *The Birth of the Clinic: An Archaeology of Medical Perception*. London: Tavistock, 1973.

———. *Discipline and Punish: The Birth of the Prison*. London: Penguin Books, 1991.

———. *History of Sexuality*. Vol. 1, *An Introduction*. London: Penguin Books, 1990.

———. 'The Politics of Health in the Eighteenth Century'. In *Power/Knowledge: Selected Interviews and Other Writings: 1972–1977*, edited by Colin Gordon. New York: Pantheon Books, 1981.

Gandhi, M.K. *Diet and Diet Reform*. Ahmedabad: Navajivan Publishing House, 1949.

———. *Hind Swaraj or Indian Home Rule*. Ahmadabad: Navajivan Publishing House, 1938.

Gangulee, N. *Health and Nutrition in India*. London: Faber and Faber, 1939.

Ghosh, Anindita. *Power in Print: Popular Publishing and the Politics of Language and Culture in a Colonial Society*. New Delhi: Oxford University Press, 2006.

Ghosh, Jajneswar. *Higher Education in Bengal under British Rule*. Calcutta: Book Company, 1926.

Ghosh, K.C. *Famines in Bengal: 1770—1943*. Calcutta: Indian Associated Publishing, 1944.

Ghosh, Suryanarayan. *Baigyanik Dampatya Pranali*. Dhaka: 1884.

Ghosh, Swati. 'Surveillance in Decolonized Social Space: The Case of Sex Workers in Bengal'. *Social Text* 23, no. 283 (Summer 2005): 55–69.

Gilman, Sander L. 'The Hottentot and the Prostitute: Towards an Iconography of Female Sexuality'. In *Difference and Pathology: Stereotypes of Sexuality, Race, and Madness*, edited by Sander L. Gilman. Ithaca: Cornell University Press, 1985.

———. *Sexuality: An Illustrated History*. New York: Wiley, 1989.

Goode, S.W. *Municipal Calcutta: Its Institutions in Their Origin and Growth*, reprint. Calcutta: Bibhash Gupta, 1916.

Gooptu, Suparna. *Cornelia Sorabji, India's Pioneer Woman Lawyer: A Biography*. New Delhi: Oxford University Press, 2006.

Gorman, Mel. 'Introduction of Western Science into Colonial India: Role of the Calcutta Medical College'. *Proceedings of the American Philosophical Society* 132, no. 3 (1988): 276–98.

Goswami, Manu. *Producing India: From Colonial Economy to National Space*. New Delhi: Permanent Black, 2004.

Greenough, Paul R. *Prosperity and Misery in Modern Bengal: The Famine of 1943–1944*. New York: Oxford University Press, 1982.

Guha, Ranajit. *Dominance without Hegemony: History and Power in Colonial India*. Cambridge, Massachusetts: Harvard University Press, 1997.

Guha, Sumit. *Health and Population in South Asia: From Earliest Times to the Present*. New Delhi: Permanent Black, 2001.

Guha, Supriya. '"The Best Swadeshi": Reproductive Health in Bengal, 1840–1940'. In Hodges, *Reproductive Health in India*.

———. 'The Unwanted Pregnancy in Colonial Bengal'. *Indian Economic and Social History Review* 33, no. 4 (1996): 403–35.

Gupta, Bramhananda. 'Indigenous Medicine in Nineteenth- and Twentieth-Century Bengal'. In Leslie, *Asian Medical Systems*, pp. 368–78.

Gupta, Charu. 'Procreation and Pleasure: Writings of a Woman Ayurvedic Practitioner in Colonial North India'. *Studies in History* 21, no. 1 (2005): 17–44.

———. *Sexuality, Obscenity, Community: Women, Muslims and the Hindu Public in Colonial India*. New Delhi: Permanent Black, 2001, second impression.

Gupta, Mohendracandra. *Stribodh*. Dacca: 1862.

Gupta, Prasannatara. *Paribarikjiban*. Calcutta: Kuntaleen Press, 1903.

Gupta, Swarupa. 'Samaj, Jati and Desh: Reflections on Nationhood in Late Colonial Bengal'. *Studies in History* 27, no. 2 (2007): 17–203.

Habib, Irfan. 'Inside and Outside the Systems: Change and Innovation in Medical and Surgical Practice in Mughal India'. In D. Kumar, *Disease and Medicine in India*.

Hall, Ruth. *Marie Stopes: A Biography*. London: Andre Deutsche Limited, 1977.

Harrison, Mark. *Climates and Constitutions: Health, Race, Environment and British Imperialism in India, 1600–1850*. New Delhi: Oxford University Press, 1999.

Harrison, Mark. 'Medicine and Orientalism: Perspectives on Europe's Encounter with Indian Medical Systems'. In *Health, Medicine and Empire: Perspectives on Colonial India*, edited by Biswamoy Pati and Mark Harrison, 37–87. New Delhi: Orient Longman, 2001.

———. *Public Health in British India: Anglo Indian Preventive Medicine, 1859–1914*. Cambridge: Cambridge University Press, 1994.

———. '"The Tender Frame of Man": Disease, Climate, and Racial Difference in India and the West Indies, 1760–1860'. *Bulletin of History of Medicine* 70 (1996): 68–93.

———. 'Tropical Medicine in Nineteenth-Century India'. *Journal of History of Science* 25 (1992): 299–318.

———. 'Towards a Sanitary Utopia? Professional Visions and Public Health in India, 1880–1914'. *South Asia Research* 10 (1990): 19–40.

Hatcher, Brian. *Idioms of Improvement: Vidyasagar and Cultural Encounter in Bengal, Delhi*. New Delhi: Oxford University Press, 1996.

Headrick, Daniel R. *The Tools of Empire: Technology and European Imperialism in the Nineteenth Century*. New York: Oxford University Press, 1981.

Hehir, Patrick. *The Medical Profession in India*. London: Oxford Medical Publishers, 1923.

Hilliker, J.F. 'The Creation of a Middle Class as a Goal of Educational Policy in Bengal 1833–1854'. In *Indian Society and the Beginnings of Modernisation, c. 1830–1850*, edited by Cyril Philips and Mary Wainwright, 31–43. London: University of London School of Oriental and African Studies, 1976.

Hochmuth, Christian. 'Patterns of Medical Culture in Colonial Bengal, 1835–1880'. *Bulletin of the History of Medicine* 80 (2006): 39–72.

Hodges, Sarah. *Conjugality, Progeny and Progress: Family and Modernity in India*. PhD diss., University of Chicago, 1999, pp. 160–208

———. 'Governmentality, Population and Reproductive Family in Modern India'. *Economic and Political Weekly* 39, no. 11 (2004): 1157–63.

———, ed. *Reproductive Health in India: History, Politics and Controversies*. Hyderabad: Orient BlackSwan, 2006.

Hyam, R. *Empire and Sexuality: The British Experience*. Manchester: Manchester University Press, 1990.

Islam, M. Mufakharul. *Bengal Agriculture, 1920–1946*. Cambridge: Cambridge University Press, 1978.

Jaggi, Om Prakash. 'Advent of English Medical Education in India'. In *Science, Philosophy and Culture: Multidisciplinary Explorations*, part I, edited by B.D. Chattopadhyaya and Ravinder Kumar, 427–64. New Delhi: The Project of History of Indian Science, Philosophy and Culture, 1996.

Jaggi, Om Prakash. *History of Science, Technology and Medicine in India*. Vol. 13, *Western Medicine in India: Medical Education and Research*. New Delhi: Atma Ram and Sons, 1979.

———. *Indian Systems of Medicine*. New Delhi: Atma Ram and Sons, 1973.

Jeffrey, P., R. Jeffrey, and A. Lyon. *Labour Pains and Labour Power: Women and Childbearing in India*. London: Zed Books, 1989.

Jeffrey, Roger. *The Politics of Health in India*. Berkley: University of California Press, 1988.

Johnson, James. *The Influence of Tropical Climates, More Especially the Climate of India on European Constitutions*. London: Stockdale, 1813.

Jolly, Julius. *Indian Medicine*, translated from German by C.G. Kashikar. New Delhi: Munshiram Manoharlal, 1994 [1951].

Jordanova, Ludmila. *Sexual Visions: Images of Gender in Science and Medicine between the Eighteenth and Twentieth Centuries*. Hemel Hempstead: Harvester Wheatsheaf, 1989.

———. 'The Social Construction of Medical Knowledge'. *Social History of Medicine* 8, no. 3 (1995): 361–81.

Kak, Shakti and Biswamoy Pati, eds. *Exploring Gender Equations: Colonial and Post Colonial India*. New Delhi: Nehru Memorial Museum and Library, 2005, pp. 93–115.

Kaminsky, Arnold P. 'Morality Legislation and British Troops in Late Nineteenth-Century India'. *Military Affairs* 43, no. 2 (1979): 78–83.

Karlekar, Malavika. 'Kadambini and the Bhadralok'. *Economic and Political Weekly* 21, no. 19 (1986): WS-25–31.

———. *Voices from Within: Early Personal Narratives of Bengali Women*. New Delhi: Oxford University Press, 1991.

Kazi, Ihtesham. 'Environmental Factors Contributing to Malaria in Colonial Bengal'. In D. Kumar, *Disease and Medicine in India*, pp. 123–31.

Khaleeli, Zhaleh. 'Harmony or Hegemony? The Rise and Fall of the Native Medical Institution, Calcutta; 1822–35'. *South Asia Research* 21 (2001): 77–104.

Khastagir, Annada Charan. *A Treatise on the Science and Practice of Midwifery with Diseases of Children and Women: Manabjanmatattwa, Dhatri Bidya, Nabaprasuta Sisu o Strijatir Byadhisangraha*, 2nd ed. Calcutta: 1878 [1868].

Kittredge, G.A. *A Short History of the 'Medical Women for India': Fund of Bombay*. Bombay: Education Society's Press, 1889.

Klein, Ira. 'Death in India'. *Journal of Asian Studies* 32 (1973): 632–59.

———. 'Malaria and Mortality in Bengal, 1840–1921'. *Indian Economic and Social History Review* 9, no. 2 (June 1972): 132–60.

Kopf, David. *The Brahmo Samaj and the Shaping of the Modern Indian Mind*. Princeton: Princeton University Press, 1979.

Kumar, Anil. *Medicine and the Raj: British Medical Policy in India, 1835–1911*. New Delhi: SAGE Publications, 1998.

Kumar, Deepak, ed. *Disease and Medicine in India: A Historical Overview*. New Delhi: Tulika, 2001.

———, ed. *Science and Empire: Essays in Indian Context (1700–1947)*. New Delhi: Anamika Prakashan, 1991.

Kumar, Neelam, ed. *Women and Science in India—A Reader*. New Delhi: Oxford University Press, 2009.

Kumar, Radha. 'Organization and Struggle'. In *History of Doing: An Illustrated Account of Movements for Women's Rights and Feminism in India 1800–1990*, edited by Radha Kumar. London: Verso, 1993.

Lal, Maneesha. '"The Politics of Gender and Medicine in Colonial India": The Countess of Dufferin's Fund, 1885–1888'. *Bulletin of the History of Medicine* 68, no. 1 (Spring 1994): 29–66.

Lang, Sean. 'Drop the Demon Dai: Maternal Mortality and the State in Colonial Madras, 1840–1875'. *Social History of Medicine* 18, no. 3 (2005): 357–78.

———. 'Obstetrics and Obstruction: Maternity Provision in Madras, 1840–1852'. In *From Western Medicine to Global Medicine: The Hospital Beyond the West*, edited by Mark Harrison, Margaret Jones, Helen Sweet, 108–41. New Delhi: Orient BlackSwan, 2009.

Legg, Stephen. 'Governing Prostitution in Colonial Delhi: From Cantonment Regulations to International Hygiene (1864–1939)'. *Social History* 34, no. 4 (2009): 447–67.

Leslie, Charles. 'Ambiguities of Revivalism in Modern India'. In Leslie, *Asian Medical Systems*, pp. 356–67.

———, ed. *Asian Medical Systems: A Comparative Study*. Berkley: University of California Press, 1976.

Levine, Philippa, ed. *Gender and Empire*. Oxford: Oxford University Press, 2004.

———. 'Orientalist Sociology and the Creation of Colonial Sexualities'. *Feminist Review* 65 (Summer 2000): 5–21.

———. *Prostitution, Race and Polities: Policing Venereal Disease in the British Empire*. London: Routledge, 2003.

———. 'Rereading the 1890s: Venereal Disease as "Constitutional Crisis" in Britain and British India'. *Journal of Asian Studies* 55, no. 3 (1996): 585–612.

———. 'Rough Usage: Prostitution, Law and the Social Historian'. In *Rethinking Social History: English Society 1570–1920 and Its Interpretation*, edited by H.N. Wilson. Manchester: Manchester University Press, 1993.

Levine, Philippa. 'Venereal Disease, Prostitution, and the Politics of Empire: The Case of British India.' *Journal of the History of Sexuality* 4 (1993–4): 579–602.

Lourdusamy, J. *Science and National Consciousness in Bengal (1870–1930)*. New Delhi: Orient Longman, 2004.

Lowe, John. *Medical Missions: Their Place and Power*. Edinburgh: Oliphant, Anderson and Ferrier, 1886.

Luke, Carmen. *Pedagogy, Printing and Protestantism: The Discourse on Childhood*. Albany: State University of New York Press, 1989.

Lushington, Charles. *The History, Design and Present State of the Religious, Benevolent and Charitable Institutions Founded by the British in Calcutta and its Vicinity*. Calcutta: Hindostanee Press, 1824.

MacKinnon, Kenneth. *A Treatise on Public Health, Climate, Hygiene and Prevailing Diseases of Bengal and the North-West Provinces*. Cawnpore: Cawnpore Press, 1848.

Mahalanobis, P.C., R. Mukherjea, and A. Ghosh. *A Sample Survey of After-effects of the Bengal Famine of 1943*. Calcutta: Statistical Publishing Society, 1946.

Maharatna, Arup. 'Infant and Child Mortality during Famines in Late 19th and Early 20th Century India.' *Economic and Political Weekly* 31, no. 27 (1996): 1774–83.

Majumdar, Baradakanta. *Naritattva*. Calcutta: 1889.

Majumdar, Pratapchandra. *Stricharitra*. Calcutta: Nababidhan, 1891.

Malhotra, Anshu. 'Of Dais and Midwives: "Middle Class" Interventions in the Management of Women's Reproductive Health in Colonial Punjab.' In Hodges, *Reproductive Health in India*, pp. 199–226.

———. *Gender, Caste, and Religious Identities*. New Delhi: Oxford University Press, 2002.

Manna, Mausumi. 'Approach towards Birth Control: Indian Women in the Early Twentieth Century.' *Indian Economic and Social History Review* 35, no. 1 (1998): 35–51.

Marks, Shula. 'What is Colonial about Colonial Medicine? And What Has Happened to Imperialism and Health?'. *Social History of Medicine* 10 (1997): 205–19.

Marston, Alice K. 'Medical Work for Women in the Mission-field.' In *Report of the Centenary Conference on the Protestant Missions of the World*, 9–19 June 1888, vol. 2, edited by J. Johnson. London: James Nisbet and Co., 1888.

Martin, James Ranald. *The Influence of Tropical Climates on European Constitutions*. London: Churchill, 1856.

———. *Notes on the Medical Topography of Calcutta*. Calcutta: Huttmann, 1837.

Mason, Michael. *The Making of Victorian Sexuality*. Oxford: Oxford University Press, 1994.

Maulitz, Russell C. *Morbid Appearances: The Anatomy of Pathology in the Early Nineteenth Century*. Cambridge: Cambridge University Press, 1987.

Mayo, Katherine. *Mother India*. London: Jonathan Cape Ltd, 1927.

McHugh, P. *Prostitution and Victorian Social Reform*. London: Croom Helm, 1980.

Metcalf, Barbara D. 'Hakim Ajmal Khan, Rais of Delhi and Muslim Leader'. In *Delhi through the Ages: Selected Essays in Urban History, Culture and Society*, edited by R.E. Frykenberg, 186–202. New Delhi: Oxford University Press, 1993.

Metcalf, Thomas R. *Ideologies of the Raj*. Vol. 3, part 4 of *The New Cambridge History of India*. Cambridge: Cambridge University Press, 1998.

Midgeley, Clare, ed. *Gender and Imperialism*. Manchester: Manchester University Press, 1998.

Mill, James. *The History of British India*, 5th ed. London: Madden, 1858.

Mills, James H. and Satadru Sen, eds. *Confronting the Body: The Politics of Physicality in Colonial and Post-colonial India*. London: Anthem Press, 2004.

Minault, Gail. *Secluded Scholars: Women's Education and Muslim Social Reform in Colonial India*. New Delhi: Oxford University Press, 1998.

Mishra, Sabyasachi R. 'An Empire "De-Masculinized": The British Colonial State and the Problem of Syphilis in Nineteenth-Century India'. In D. Kumar, *Disease and Medicine in India*, pp. 166–79.

Mitra, Durgadas. 'Diet and Nutrition of Bengali Hindus'. *Indian Medical Gazette*, April 1939.

Mitra, Lilabati. 'Grihaswasthye Ramanir Dristi'. *Antahpur* 7 (1905): 9.

Mitra, R.C. 'Education'. In Sinha, *History of Bengal*.

Moore, W. *A Manual of Family Medicine for India*, 2nd edition. London: Churchill, 1877.

Mukerjee, Madhusree. *Churchill's Secret War: The British Empire and the Ravaging of India during World War II*. New York: Basic Books, 2010.

Mukerji, Karunamoy. *Agriculture, Famine and Rehabilitation in South Asia*. Santiniketan: Visva Bharati, 1965.

Mukharji, Projit Bihari. *Nationalizing the Body: The Medical Market, Print and Daktari Medicine*. London: Anthem Press, 2009.

Mukherjee, Malavika. *The Famine of 1896–1897 in Bengal: Availability or Entitlement Crisis?* New Delhi: Orient Longman, 2004.

Mukherjee, Radhakamal. *The Changing Face of Bengal: A Study in the Riverine Economy*, reprint. Calcutta: University of Calcutta, 2008–9.

Mukherjee, Sujata. 'Disciplining the Body? Health Care for Women and Children in Early Twentieth Century Bengal'. In D. Kumar, *Disease and Medicine in India*.

Mukherjee, Sujata. 'Environmental Thoughts and Malaria in Colonial Bengal: A Study in Social Response'. *Economic and Political Weekly* 43, nos 12–13 (2008): 54–61.

———. 'Imperialism, Medicine and Women's Health in Nineteenth Century India'. In *Science and Society in India, c. 1750–2000*, edited by Arun Bandopadhyay, 95–120. New Delhi: Manohar, 2010.

———. 'Malaria and Morbidity in Colonial Bengal'. In *The Imperial Embrace: Society and Polity under the Raj: Essays in Honour of Sunil Kumar Sen*, edited by Ranjit Kumar Roy. Calcutta: Rabindra Bharati University, 1993.

———. 'Medical Education and the Emergence of Women Medics in Colonial Bengal'. Occasional Paper 37, Institute of Development Studies Kolkata (2012).

———. 'Women and Medicine in Colonial India: A Case Study of Three Women Doctors'. *Indian History Congress Proceedings*, 66th session, 2005–6, pp. 1184–91.

———. 'Women, Medicine and Empire: Female Practitioners and Patterns of Health Care in Colonial Bengal'. *Modern Historical Studies* 2 (2001): 187–204.

Mukhopadhyaya, Bipradas. *Yuvak-yuvati*. Calcutta: 1922 [1891].

Mukhopadhyaya, Gangaprasad. *Matrishiksha*. Calcutta: United Press, 1902.

Mukhopadhyaya, Girindranath. *History of Indian Medicine from the Earliest Ages to the Present Time*, 2 vols. Calcutta: University of Calcutta, 1923.

Mukhopadhyaya, Jadunath. *Dhatrishiksha evam Prasutishiksha Arthat Kkathopakathanchhale Dhai evam Prasutidiger Prati Upadesh*. Chinsura: Chikitsabodhak Press, 1875 [1867].

Mullens, Hannah Catherine. 'Phulmani o Karunar Bibaran'. In *Women Writing in India*, vol. 1, *600 BC to the Present*, edited by Susie Tharu and K. Lalitha, 205. New York: Feminist Press, 1991.

Muraleedharan, V.R. 'Malady in Madras: The Colonial Government's Response to Malaria in the Early Twentieth Century'. In D. Kumar, *Science and Empire*.

Murshid, Ghulum. *Reluctant Debutante: Response of Bengali Women to Modernization, 1849–1905*. Rajshahi: Rajshahi University Press, 1983.

Nag, Kalidas, ed. *Bethune College and School, Centenary Volume, 1849–1949*. Calcutta: Saraswati Press, 1950.

Nair, Janaki. 'Uncovering the Zenana: Visions of Indian Womanhood in Englishwomen's Writings, 1813–1940'. *Journal of Women's History* 2, no. 11 (Spring 1990): 8–34.

———. *Women and Law in Colonial India: A Social History*. New Delhi and Bangalore: Kali for Women and National Law School of India University, 1996.

Nandy, Ashis. *The Intimate Enemy: Loss and Recovery of Self under Colonialism*. New Delhi: Oxford University Press, 1983.

Nandy, Ashis. 'The Psychology of Colonialism: Sex, Age and Ideology in British India'. *Psychiatry* 45 (1982): 197–218.

Narayan, T.G. *Famine over Bengal*. Calcutta: The Book Company Limited, 1944.

Neelameghan, A. *The Development of Medical Societies and Medical Periodicals in India, 1780 to 1920*. Calcutta: Indian Association of Special Libraries and Information Centres, 1963.'I

Nicholas, R.W. 'The Goddess Sitala and Epidemic Smallpox in Bengal'. *Journal of Asian Studies* 41, no. 1 (1981): 21–44.

Nutton, Vivian. 'Humoralism'. In *Companion Encyclopedia of the History of Medicine*, edited by W.F. Bynum and Porter Roy. London: Routledge, 1993.

Ogborn, Miles. 'Law and Discipline in Nineteenth Century English State Formation: The Contagious Diseases Acts of 1864, 1866, and 1869'. *Journal of Historical Sociology* 6, no. 1 (March 1993): 28–55.

Orme, Robert. *Government and the People of Indostan*, part I. Lucknow: Pustak Kendra, 1971 [1753].

Pachauri, S., ed. *Implementing a Reproductive Health Agenda in India: The Beginning: South and South-East Asia*. Population Council, 1999.

Palit, Chittabrata and Achintya Kumar Dutta, eds. *History of Medicine in India: The Medical Encounter*. New Delhi: Kalpaz Publications, 2005.

Pande, Ishita. *Medicine, Race and Liberalism in British Bengal: Symptoms of Empire*. London and New York: Routledge, 2010.

Panikkar, K.N. *Culture, Ideology, Hegemony: Intellectuals and Social Consciousness in Colonial India*. New Delhi: Tulika, 2001.

Parulekar, R.V. *Survey of Indigenous Education in the Madras Presidency, 1822–26*. Reprinted in *The Beautiful Tree*, edited by Dharampal. New Delhi: Biblia Impex Pvt. Ltd, 1983.

———. *Survey of Indigenous Education in the Province of Bombay, 1820–30*. Bombay: Asia Publishing House, 1951.

Peers, Douglas M. 'Soldiers, Surgeons and the Campaigns to Combat Sexually Transmitted Diseases in Colonial India, 1805–1860', *Medical History* 42, no. 2 (1998): 137–60.

———. 'War and Public Finance in Early Nineteenth-Century British India: the First Burma War'. *International History Review* 11 (1989): 628–47.

Philips, Richard. 'Imperialism, Sexuality and Space: Purity Movements in the British Empire'. In *Postcolonial Geographies*, edited by A. Blunt and C. McEwan. New York, London: Continuum, 2002.

Porter, Roy. 'Hospitals and Surgery'. In *The Cambridge History of Medicine*, edited by Roy Porter. New York: Cambridge University Press, 2006.

Porter, Roy and Lesley Hall. *The Facts of Life: The Creation of Sexual Knowledge in Britain, 1650–1950*. New Haven: Yale University Press, 1995.

Powell, Avril A. and Siobhan Lambert-Hurley, eds. *Rhetoric and Reality: Gender and the Colonial Experience in South Asia*. New Delhi: Oxford University Press, 2006.

Prakash, Gyan. *Another Reason: Science and the Imagination of Modern India*. Princeton: Princeton University Press, 1999.

———. 'Science between the Lines'. In *Subaltern Studies IX*, edited by Shahid Amin and Dipesh Chakrabarty. New Delhi: Oxford University Press, 1996.

'Presidential Address of Dr. B.C. Roy, All India Medical Conference, Lahore, December 1929'. *Journal of the Indian Medical Association* 1, no. 1 (March 1930): 3–4.

Procida, Mary. *Married to the Empire: Gender, Politics and Imperialism in India, 1883–1947*. Manchester and New York: Manchester University Press, 2002.

Raha, Bipasha. *The Plough and the Pen: Peasantry, Agriculture and the Literati in Colonial Bengal*. New Delhi: Manohar, 2012.

Raj, Kapil, 'Knowledge, Power and Modern Science: The Brahmins Strike Back'. In D. Kumar, *Science and Empire*.

Rajwade, Laxmibai. 'Indian Mother'. In *Our Cause: A Symposium by Indian Women*, edited by Shyam Kumari Nehru. Allahabad: Kitabistan, n.d.

Ramanna, Mridula. 'Control and Resistance: The Working of the Contagious Diseases Acts in Bombay City'. *Economic And Political Weekly* 35, no. 17 (2000): 1470–6.

———. *Health Care in Bombay Presidency: 1896–1930*. New Delhi: Primus Books, 2012.

Ramasubban, Radhika. 'Imperial Health in British India, 1857–1900'. In *Disease, Medicine and Empire: Perspectives on Western Medicine and the Experience of European Expansion*, edited by Roy Macleod and Milton Lewis, 38–60. London: Routledge, 1988.

———. 'Public Health and Medical Research in India: Their Origins under the Impact of British Colonial Policy'. *SAREC Report*. Stockholm: 1982.

Ramusack, Barbara N. 'Cultural Missionaries, Maternal Imperialists: Feminist Allies: British Women Activists in India, 1865–1945'. In N. Choudhuri and Strobel, *Western Women and Imperialism*, pp. 119–36.

———. 'Embattled Advocates: The Debate over Birth Control in India, 1920–1940'. *Journal of Women's History* 1, no. 2 (1989): 34–64.

———. 'Women's Organizations and Social Change: The Age-of-marriage Issue in India'. In *Women and World Change: Equity Issues in Development*, edited by Naomi Black and Ann Baker Cottrell, 198–216. Beverly Hills, California: SAGE Publications, 1981.

Rao, Mohan. *From Population Control to Reproductive Health: Malthusian Arithmetic*. New Delhi: SAGE Publications, 2004.

Rassundari Devi. 'Amar Jiban'. In *Atmakatha*, edited by Nareshchandra Jana, Manu Jana, and Kamalkumar Sanyal, vol. 1. Calcutta: Ananya Prakashan, 1981.

Ray, Kabita. *History of Public Health: Colonial Bengal 1921–1947*. Calcutta: K.P. Bagchi & Company, 1998.

Ray, Kumudini. 'Hindu Narir Garhasthyadharmma'. *Bamabodhini Patrika* 5, no. 3 (1894).

Ray, Rajat Kanta. *Felt Community: Community and Mentality before the Emergence of Indian Nationalism*. New Delhi: Oxford University Press, 2003.

Ray, Sibnarayan. *Bengal Renaissance: The First Phase*. Calcutta: Minerva Associates, 2000.

Ray, Utsa. *Culinary Culture in Colonial India: A Cosmopolitan Platter and the Middle-Class*. New Delhi: Cambridge University Press, 2015.

Raychaudhuri, Tapan. *Europe Reconsidered: Perceptions of the West in Nineteenth-Century Bengal*. New Delhi: Oxford University Press, 1988.

———. 'The Pursuit of Reason in Nineteenth-Century Bengal'. In *Perceptions, Emotions, Sensibilities: Essays on India's Colonial and Post-Colonial Experiences*, edited by Tapan Raychaudhuri, 49–65. New Delhi: Oxford University Press, 1999.

Richards, Frank. *Old Soldier Sahib*. London: Faber and Faber, 1936.

Ridsdale, W. *Record of Cases Treated in the Mesmeric Hospital—From June to December, 1847*. Calcutta, Military Orphan Press, 1848.

Roberton, John. *Essays and Notes on the Physiology and Diseases of Women, and on Practical Midwifery*. London: John Churchill, 1851.

Rosselli, John. 'The Self-Image of Effeteness: Physical Education and Nationalism in Nineteenth-Century Bengal'. *Past and Present* 87 (February 1980): 121–48.

Roychowdhury, Deboshruti. *Gender and Caste Hierarchy in Colonial Bengal: Inter-Caste Interventions of Ideal Womanhood*. Kolkata: Stree, 2014.

Said, Edward W. *Culture And Imperialism*. New York: Vintage Books, 1994.

Samanta, Arabinda. *Malarial Fever in Colonial Bengal, 1820–1939: Social History of an Epidemic*. Calcutta: Firma KLM Private Limited, 2002.

———. 'Physicians, Forceps and Childbirth: Technological Intervention in Reproductive Health in Colonial Bengal'. In *Medicine and Colonialism: Historical Perspectives in India and South Africa*, edited by Poonam Bala, 111–26. London: Pickering & Chatto, 2014.

Sangari, Kumkum and Sudesh Vaid, eds. *Recasting Women: Essays in Indian Colonial History*. New Brunswick, New Jersey: Rutgers University Press, 1990.

Sarkar, Mahendra Lal. *A Sketch of the Treatment of Cholera*. Kolkata: Anglo Sanskrit Press, 1904 [1870].

Sarkar, Sumit. *Writing Social History*. New Delhi, New York: Oxford University Press, 1997.

Sarkar, Tanika. *Hindu Wife, Hindu Nation: Community, Religion, and Cultural Nationalism*. Bloomington: Indiana University Press, 2001.

———. *Words to Win: The Making of Amar Jiban, a Modern Autobiography*. New Delhi: Kali for Women, 1999.

Sastri, Sivnath. *History of the Brahmo Samaj*, 2nd ed. Calcutta: Brahmo Mission Press, 1974.

Sawday, Jonathan. *The Body Emblazoned: Dissection and the Human Body in Renaissance Culture*. London: Routledge, 1995.

Scharlieb, Mary. *Reminiscences*. London: Williams and Norgate, 1924.

Sehrawat, Samikhsha. *Colonial Medical Care in North India: Gender, State, and Society, c. 1840–1920*. New Delhi: Oxford University Press, 2013.

———. 'The Foundation of the Lady Hardinge Medical College and Hospital for Women at Delhi: Issues in Women's Medical Education and Imperial Governance'. In Kak and Pati, *Exploring Gender Equations*, pp. 117–46.

Sen, Amartya. 'Famine Mortality: A Study of the Bengal Famine of 1943'. In *Peasants in History: Essays in Honour of Daniel Thorner*, edited by E.J. Hobsbawm, W. Kula, A. Mitra, K. N. Raj and I. Sachs, 194–220. Calcutta: Oxford University Press, 1980.

———. *Poverty and Famines: An Essay on Entitlement and Deprivation*. New Delhi: Oxford University Press, 1984.

Sen, Asok, Partha Chatterjee, and Saugata Mukherji, eds. *Three Studies on the Agrarian Structure in Bengal, 1840–1947*. New Delhi: Oxford University Press, 1982.

Sen, Bhowani. *Rural Bengal in Ruins*, translated by N. Chakravarty. Bombay: People's Publishing House, 1945.

Sen, Dinescandra. *Gribasri*. Calcutta: 1915.

Sen, Indrani. 'The Memsahib's "Madness": The European Woman's Mental Health in Late Nineteenth Century India'. *Social Scientist* 33, vol. 5–6 (2005): 26–48.

———. 'Resisting Patriarchy: Complexities and Conflicts in the Memoir of Haimabati Sen'. *Economic and Political Weekly* 47, no. 12 (2012): 55–62.

Sen, S.N. *Scientific and Technical Education in India 1781–1900*. New Delhi: Indian National Science Academy, 1991.

Sen, Samita. *Women and Labour in Late Colonial India: The Bengal Jute Industry*. Cambridge: Cambridge University Press, 1999.

Sen, Samita and Anirban Das. 'A History of the Calcutta Medical College and Hospital, 1835–1936'. In *Science and Modern India: An Institutional History, c. 1784–1947*, edited by Uma Dasgupta, 477–522. Vol. 15, part IV of *Project of History of Science, Philosophy and Culture in Indian Civilization*. New Delhi: Pearson Publishers, 2011.

Seton-Karr, W.S. *Selections from Calcutta Gazettes*, vol. 2. Calcutta: O.T. Cutter, Military Orphan Press, 1865.

Sharma, Madhuri. '*Debating Women's Health: Reflections in Popular Hindi Print-culture*'. *Indian Historical Review* 35, vol. II: 178–90.

———. *Indigenous and Western Medicine in Colonial India*. New Delhi: Foundation Books, 2012.

Sharp, H., ed. *Progress of Education in India: 1907–1912. Sixth Quinquennial Review*, vol. 1. Calcutta: 1914, pp. 151–2.

Sigerist, Henry E. *Civilization and Disease*. Chicago: University of Chicago Press, 1962.

Singh, Dhrub Kumar. 'Cholera: Changing Perceptions of its Causality in the Last Two Centuries–A Cursory Appraisal'. In Palit and A.K. Dutta, *History of Medicine in India*, pp. 67–86.

Singh, Maina Chawla. 'Gender, Medicine and Empire: Early Initiatives in Institution Building and Professionalisation (1890s–1940s)'. In Kak and Pati, *Exploring Gender Equations*, pp. 93–115.

———. *Gender, Religion and 'Heathen Lands': American Missionary Women in South Asia (1860–1940s)*. New York: Garland, 2000.

Sinha, J.N. 'Science and the Indian National Congress'. In D. Kumar, *Science and Empire*, pp. 161–81.

Sinha, Mrinalini. *Colonial Masculinity: The 'Manly Englishman' and the 'Effeminate Bengali' in the Late Nineteenth Century*. New York: Manchester University Press, 1995.

———. 'Lineage of the "Indian" Modern: Rhetoric, Agency and the Sarda Act in Late Colonial India'. In *Gender, Sexuality and Colonial Modernity*, edited by Antoinette Burton, 207–21. London: Routledge, 2000.

Sinha, N.K., ed. *History of Bengal, 1757–1905*, 2nd ed. Calcutta: University of Calcutta, 1996.

Sinha, Sandip. *Public Health Policy and the Indian Public: Bengal 1850–1920*. Calcutta: Vision Publications, 1998.

Sivaramakrishnan, Kavita. *Old Potions, New Bottles: Recasting Indigenous Medicine in Colonial Punjab (1850–1945)*. Hyderabad: Orient Longman, 2006.

Smith, F.B. 'The Contagious Diseases Acts Reconsidered'. *Social History of Medicine* 3, no. 2 (1990): 197–215.

Smith, F.B. 'Ethics and Disease in the Later Nineteenth Century: The Contagious Diseases Acts'. *Historical Studies* 15, (1971): 118–35.

Smith, F.B. *The People's Health: 1830–1910*. London: Croom Helm, 1979, p. 114. In Guha, *Health and Population in South Asia*.

Spiers, Edward M. *The Army and the Society 1815–1914*. London: Longman, 1980.

Srimanjari. *Through War and Famine: Bengal, 1939–45*. New Delhi: Orient BlackSwan, 2009.

Stoler, Ann Laura. *Race and the Education of Desire: Foucault's History of Sexuality and the Colonial Order of Things*. Durham, North Carolina and London: Duke University Press, 1995.

Subramaniam, Lakshmi. 'The Master, Muse, and the Nation'. *South Asia* 23, no. 2 (2000): 1–32.

Sundara Raj, M. *Prostitution in Madras: A Study in Historical Perspective*. New Delhi: Konark Publications Pvt. Ltd, 1993.

Twinning, William. *Clinical Illustrations of the More Important Diseases of Bengal with the Results of an Enquiry into Their Pathology and Treatment*, 2 vols, 2nd edition. Calcutta: Mission Press, 1835.

Vaughan, Megan. *Curing Their Ills: Colonial Power and African Illness*. Stanford: Stanford University Press, 1991.

Visaria, Leela and Pradip Visaria. 'Population'. In *Cambridge Economic History of India*, vol. 2, *c. 1757 to c. 1970*, edited by Dharma Kumar and Meghnad Desai, 463–532. New Delhi: Orient Longman, 1982.

Walkowitz, Judith R. *Prostitution and Victorian Society: Women, Class, and the State*. Cambridge: Cambridge University Press, 1980.

Walsh, Judith E. *How to Be the Goddess of Your Home: An Anthology of Bengali Domestic Manuals*. New Delhi: Yoda Press, 2005.

Ward, William. *A View of the History, Literature and Mythology of the Hindoos Including a Minute Description of Their Manners and Customs*. Serampore: Mission Press, 1818.

Webb, Allen. *Pathologica Indica, or, the Anatomy of Indian Diseases, Medical and Surgical: Based upon Morbid Specimens from All Parts of India in the Museum of the Calcutta Medical College; Illustrated by Detailed Cases, with the Prescriptions and Treatment Employed, and Comments, Physiological, Practical and Historical*, 2nd edition. London: W.H. Allen and Co., 1848.

Weeks, Jeffrey. *Sex, Politics and Society: The Regulation of Sexuality since 1800*, 2nd edition. UK: Pearson Education Ltd, 1989.

Werth, Paul. 'Through the Prism of Prostitution: State, Society and Power', *Social History* 1, vol. 19 (1994): 1–15.

Whitehead, Judy. 'Bodies Clean and Unclean: Prostitution, Sanitary Legislation and Respectable Femininity in Colonial North India.' *Gender and History* 7, no. 1 (1995): 41–63.

———. 'Modernising the Motherhood Archetype: Public Health Models and the Child Marriage Restraint Act of 1929'. In *Social Reform, Sexuality and the State*, edited by Patricia Uberoi, 188–209. New Delhi: SAGE Publications, 1996.

Williamson, Captain Thomas. *East India Vade-Mecum*, vol. 2. London: Black, Parry and Kingsbury, 1810.

Wise, James. *Notes on the Races, Castes and Tribes of Eastern Bengal*. Unpublished.

Wise, T.A. *Commentary on the Hindu System of Medicine*, 2nd ed. London: Trubner and Co., 1860.

Worboys, Michael. 'The Discovery of Colonial Malnutrition between the Wars'. In *Imperial Medicine and Indigenous Societies*, edited by David Arnold, 208–25. Manchester: Manchester University Press, 1988.

Wujastyk, Dominik. *The Roots of Ayurveda: Selections from Sanskrit Medical Writings*. New Delhi: Penguin, 1998.

Wyke, T.J. 'Hospital Facilities For, and Diagnosis and Treatment of, Venereal Disease in England, 1800–1870'. *British Journal of Venereal Diseases* 49, no. 1 (1973): 78–85.

———. 'The Manchester and Salford Lock Hospital, 1818–1917'. *Medical History* 19 (1975): 73–86.

Young, Ruth. 'Medical Women and Contraception Control'. *Journal of Association of Medical Women in India* 22, no. 2 (1934): 5–12.

Zimmermann, Francis. *The Jungle and the Aroma of Meats: An Ecological Theme in Hindu Medicine*. Berkeley: University of California Press, 1987.

Index

About the Author

Sujata Mukherjee is Professor, Department of History, and Dean of Arts Faculty, Rabindra Bharati University, Kolkata. She was the ICCR Visiting Chair at Victoria University, Wellington, New Zealand, between July and October 2016.